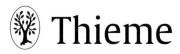

# ıe Chest X-Ray

## Differential Diagnosis in Conventional Radiology

Francis A. Burgener, M.D.
Professor of Radiology
University of Rochester
Medical Center
Rochester, N.Y., U.S.A.

Martti Kormano, M.D.
Formerly Professor and Chairman
Department of Radiology
University of Turku
Turku, Finland

Tomi Pudas, M.D.
Department of Radiology
University of Turku
Turku, Finland

2nd revised edition

498 illustrations

Thieme
Stuttgart · New York

*Library of Congress Cataloging-in-Publication Data*
is available from the publisher.

**Important Note:** Medicine is an ever-changing science undergoing continual development. Research and clinical experience are continually expanding our knowledge, in particular our knowledge of proper treatment and drug therapy. Insofar as this book mentions any dosage or application, readers may rest assured that the authors, editors and publishers have made every effort to ensure that such references are in accordance **with the state of knowledge at the time of production of the book.**

Nevertheless this does not involve, imply, or express any guarantee or responsibility on the part of the publishers in respect of any dosage instructions and forms of application stated in the book. **Every user is requested to examine** carefully the manufacturers' leaflets accompanying each drug and to check, if necessary in consultation with a physician or specialist, whether the dosage schedules mentioned therein or the contraindications stated by the manufacturers differ from the statements made in the present book. Such examination is particularly important with drugs that are either rarely used or have been newly released on the market. **Every dosage schedule or every form of application used is entirely at the user's own risk and responsibility.** The authors and publishers request every user to report to the publishers any discrepancies or inaccuracies noticed.

© 2006 Georg Thieme Verlag,
Rüdigerstraße 14, D-70469 Stuttgart, Germany
http://www.thieme.de

Thieme New York, 333 Seventh Avenue,
New York, N.Y. 10001, U.S.A
http://www.thieme.de

Cover design: Martina Berge, Erbach
Typesetting by primustype Hurler GmbH,
D-73274 Notzingen
Printed in Germany by Grammlich, Pliezhausen

ISBN 3-13-107612-7 (GTV, Stuttgart)
ISBN 1-58890-446-6 (TMP, New York)          1 2 3 4 5

Some of the product names, patents and registered designs referred to in this book are in fact registered trademarks or proprietary names even though specific reference to this fact is not always made in the text. Therefore, the appearance of a name without designation as proprietary is not to be construed as a representation by the publisher that it is in the public domain.

# Preface

Conventional radiography remains the backbone in thoracic radiology despite the advent of newer and more exciting imaging techniques such as computed tomography, high resolution computed tomography, magnetic resonance imaging and most recently positron emission tomography. In contrast to many of these newer methods, conventional radiography is practiced not only by radiologists but also by a large number clinicians and surgeons. With each examination, one is confronted with radiologic findings that require interpretation in order to arrive at a general diagnostic impression and a reasonable differential diagnosis. To assist the film reader in attaining this goal this book is based upon radiographic finding unlike most other textbooks in radiology that are disease oriented. Since many diseases present radiographically in a varicty of manifestations some overlap in the text is unavoidable. To minimize repetition the differential diagnosis of a radiographic findings is presented in tabular form whenever feasible. Most tables do not only list the various diseases that may present radiologically in a specific pattern, but also describe in succinct form other characteristically associated radiographic findings and pertinent clinical data. Radiographic illustrations and drawings are included to demonstrate visually the radiographic features under discussion.

The transition from film to digital radiography had the greatest impact on conventional radiology since the publication of the last edition. This change however did not affect the way radiologic diagnoses are ascertained. Since the publication of the last edition in 1992 the name of a few disorders has changed (e. g., histiocytosis X to Langerhans cell histiocytosis) and a few disease are newly recognized (e. g. severe acute respiratory distress syndrome or SARS). These facts were taken into account in the new edition. The text was updated, many illustrations replaced and large numbers of new illustrations added.

A changing of the guard has also taken place. Since Dr. Martti Kormano's professional endeavors do no longer include clinical radiology, he felt no longer up to the task to update his original contributions to the text. He was however very fortunate to find in Dr. Tomi Pudas a very talented young radiologist to take over the revision of the chapters originally prepared by him.

I hope this new edition will be as well received as its predecessors in the past that produced several spin-off books and were translated into five foreign languages. The concept of an imaging pattern approach in tabular form rather than a disease oriented text was introduced in 1985 with the original edition and has since been adopted by many authors. I feel complimented by the old cliché, "imitation is the sincerest form of flattery."

This book is meant for physicians with some experience in chest radiology who wish to strengthen their diagnostic acumen. It is a comprehensive outline of radiographic findings and it should be particularity useful to radiology residents preparing for their specialist examinations, especially since the exposure to conventional radiography during their training continuously decreased in the past in favor of newer imaging modalities. Any physician involved in the interpretation of conventional chest radiograph examinations should find this book helpful in direct proportion to his curiosity.

It is my hope that this new edition will be as well received as the previous ones by medical students, residents, radiologists and physicians involved in the interpretation of conventional chest radiographs were.

*Francis A. Burgener, M.D.*

# Acknowledgements

It is impossible to thank individually all those who helped to prepare the third edition of this textbook. I wish to acknowledge the staff of Thieme, in particular Dr. Clifford Bergman and Mr. Gert A. Krüger.

I am deeply indebted to Dr. Gertrud Gollman, Steinach am Attersee, Austria, who translated the last edition of this text into German and suggested many alterations and corrections, which have been incorporated into this new edition.

My gratitude goes to all the radiologists whose cooperation made available illustrative cases to compliment the original collection or to replace older illustrations. I am indebted to Drs. Steven P. Meyers, Johnny U. V. Monu, and Gwy Suk Seo, all staff members of the University of Rochester Radiology Department, and to the former residents Drs. John M. Fitzgerald and Wael E. A. Saad for providing selected cases.

I wish to express also many thanks to Jeanette Griebel, Iona Mackey, and Marcella Maier for their assistance in preparing the references and to Shirley Cappiello for her general assistance. Last, but not least, I am most grateful to Alyce Norder who left the University and me after 30 years for the richness of the industry. She is the only person capable of deciphering my longhand and, as in the past, did a superb job in typing, editing, and proofreading the manuscript of the new edition of this text. Despite her heavy workload as executive assistant in her new endeavor. Alyce was kind enough to perform this task in her spare time, for which I am greatly appreciative.

Finally I appreciate the support of my wife Therese, who has generously given her precious family time for the preparation of this book.

*Francis A. Burgener, M.D.*

I would like to express my deepest gratitude to honorary professor Martti Kormano who invited me to carry on his work in this new edition. I continue to admire the massive work that he and Dr. Burgener originally put into the project in the early nineteen-eighties. The hundreds of hours which Dr. Kormano and I have spent together editing this edition have been a great pleasure. It was a fascinating time in my life.

I especially want to thank Drs. Kimmo Mattila and Seppo Koskinen for introducing me to musculoskeletal radiology, and for their extraordinary teaching and support. Many thanks also belong to Drs. Erkki Svedström, Risto Elo, and Peter B. Dean for encouraging me on my way in the field of radiology. The many fascinating discussions I have had with Drs. Seppo Kortelainen and Teemu Paavilainen brought me much delight, on non-radiological topics as much as on professional subjects.

I also express sincere thanks to the staff of the publishers, Thieme, especially to Dr. Clifford Bergman and Mr. Gert Krüger. Finally, much gratitude is due to Mr. Markku Livanaien for his valuable assistance with technical questions, and to Ms. Pirjo Helanko for all her help with general matters. Many other individuals helped in various ways with this project, and though I cannot name them all, I am grateful for their contributions.

*Tomi Pudas, M.D.*

# Contents

# Abbreviations

| | |
|---|---|
| ACTH | adrenocorticotropic hormone |
| AIDS | acquired immune deficiency syndrome |
| ALL | acute lymphoblastic leukemia |
| AML | acute myeloblastic leukemia |
| ANCA | antineutrophil cytoplasmotic autoantibodies |
| ANT | anterior |
| AP | anteroposterior |
| APVR | anomalous pulmonary venous return |
| ARDS | acute respiratory distress syndrome |
| ATN | acute tubular necrosis |
| AV | arteriovenous |
| AVF | arteriovenous fistula |
| AVM | arteriovenous malformation |
| AVN | avascular necrosis |
| Bx | biopsy |
| CAD | coronary artery disease |
| CAM | cystic adenomatoid malformation |
| CHF | congestive heart failure |
| CID | cytomegalic inclusion disease |
| CLL | chronic lymphatic leukemia |
| CMV | cytomegalovirus |
| CNS | central nervous system |
| COPD | chronic obstructive pulmonary disease |
| CT | computed tomography |
| DD | differential diagnosis |
| DIC | dissemination intravascular coagulation |
| DIP | desquamative interstitial pneumonitis |
| EG | eosinophilic granuloma |
| F | female |
| GE | gastroesophageal |
| GIP | giant cell interstitial pneumonitis |
| Hb | hemoglobin |
| HD | Hodgkin disease |
| HIV | human immunodeficiency virus |
| HRCT | high-resolution CT |
| Hx | history |
| IM | intramuscular |
| IVC | inferior vena cava |
| L | left |
| LA | left atrium |
| LCH | Langerhans cell histiocytosis |
| LE | lupus erythematosus |
| LIP | lymphoid interstitial pneumonitis |
| LL | lower lobes |
| LLL | left lower lobe |
| LLQ | left lower quadrant |
| LUL | left upper lobe |
| LUQ | left upper quadrant |
| LV | left ventricle |
| M | male |
| MAI | Mycobacterium avium intracellulare |
| MFH | malignant fibrous histiocytoma |
| ML | middle lobe |
| MPS | mucopolysaccharidosis |
| MR | magnetic resonance |
| MRI | magnetic resonance imaging |
| NHL | non-Hodgkin lymphoma |
| NUC | nuclear medicine |
| PA | posteroanterior |
| PAPVR | partial anomalous pulmonary venous return |
| PATH | pathology |
| PAVM | pulmonary arteriovenous malformation |
| PCP | Pneumocystis carinii pneumonia |
| PDA | patent ductus arteriosus |
| PE | pulmonary embolism |
| PET | positron emission tomography |
| PNET | primitive neuroectodermal tumor |
| PO | per oral |
| RA | rheumatoid arthritis |
| RA | right atrium |
| RBC | red blood cell |
| RDS | respiratory distress syndrome |
| RES | reticuloendothelial system |
| RLL | right lower lobe |
| RLQ | right lower quadrant |
| RML | right middle lobe |
| RUL | right upper lobe |
| RV | right ventricle |
| SARS | severe acute respiratory distress syndrome |
| SLE | systemic lupus erythematosus |
| TAPVR | total anomalous pulmonary venous return |
| TB | tuberculosis |
| TNM | tumor-node-metastasis |
| UIP | usual interstitial pneumonitis |
| US | ultrasound |

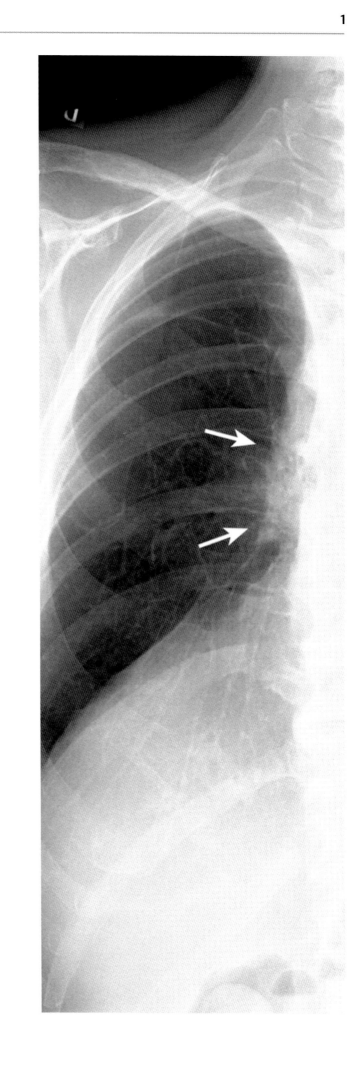

# 1 Cardiac Enlargement

Most of the diseases involving the heart will cause either generalized or localized enlargement of the heart or great vessels. A small heart is usually constitutional (asthenia, senility, wasting) and only rarely reflects a disease (Fig. 1.1). Exceptions to this are *adrenal insufficiency, constrictive pericarditis, dehydration*, or an *asthmatic paroxysm* with emphysema, where a relatively small heart may be considered to reflect the effects of the disease process itself.

The size of the heart can be estimated in several ways. A simple approach is the *cardiothoracic index*: the ratio between the total transverse diameter of the cardiac shadow and the internal diameter of the chest (Fig. 1.1 a). After the age of 5 years, this ratio normally varies, between 0.4 and 0.5. In smaller children and neonates, the ratio may be as high as 0.6, and during the second month after birth even 0.65.

The cardiac volume can be estimated with a fair degree of accuracy by measuring the *relative volume* of the heart according to the following equation:

$$\text{Relative cardiac volume} = \frac{L \times B \times S \times 0.44}{\text{body surface area (m}^2)}$$

where L = longest diameter of the heart in posteroanterior view; B = broad diameter of the heart (perpendicular to L); and S = longest sagittal diameter of the heart in lateral view (Fig. 1.1 b, c). Factor 0.44 applies to the film-focus distance of 2 m. If this distance is 1.5 m, a factor of 0.42 should be used instead. The surface area of the body is available from charts if the height and weight of the body are known (Fig. 1.2). The relative volume of the heart shows great interindividual variation. Values between 350 cc/m$^2$ and 500 cc/m$^2$ are considered normal for men. In women they tend to be slightly smaller. A single measurement of the relative volume has therefore little diagnostic value, but it may be useful in the follow-up of an individual patient, since many interindividual variables are then excluded. Interindividual variation of interthoracic pressure and other factors still have a great effect (Fig. 1.3). Enlargement of individual chambers of

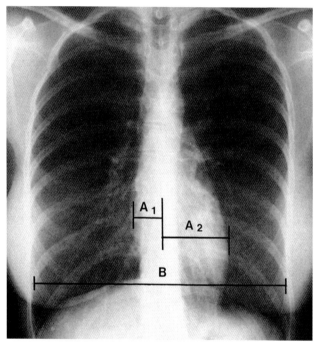

a

Fig. 1.**1 a**   Small heart in an asthenic woman, age 20. The method of measuring the cardiothoracic index is shown.

$$\text{Cardiothoracic index} = \frac{(A1 + A2)}{B}$$

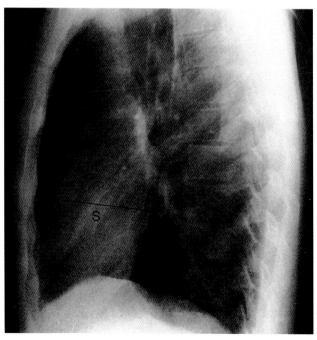

b

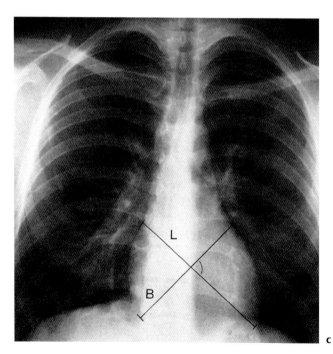

c

Fig. 1.**1 b, c**

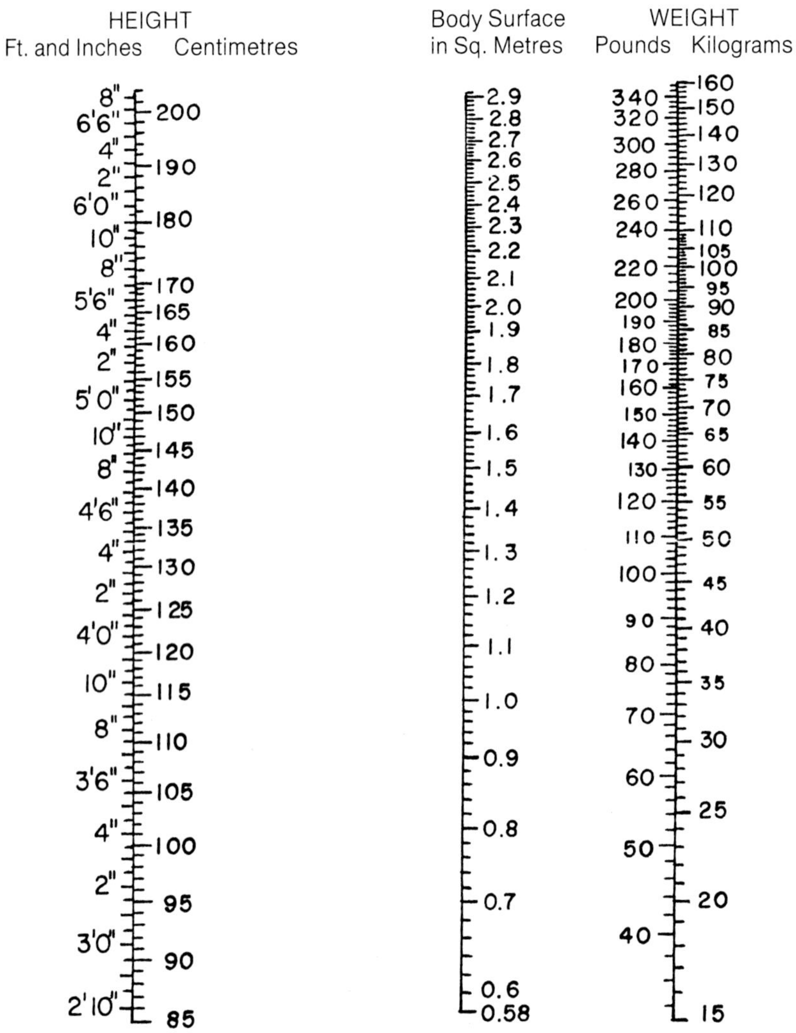

HEIGHT
Ft. and Inches    Centimetres

Body Surface
in Sq. Metres

WEIGHT
Pounds  Kilograms

Fig. 1.2  Nomogram for the determination of body surface area of adults (adapted from Documenta Geigy, Scientific Tables, Basel). Join patients weight and weight with a line. In the mid column you find the body surface.

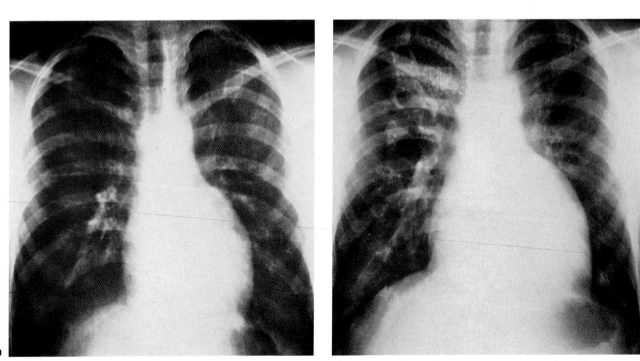

**a**    **b**

Fig. 1.3  Great change in the appearance of heart size is produced by the Valsalva effect. The two exposures were taken a few minutes apart.

the heart may cause typical configurations, as seen in Fig. 1.**4**. When there is enlargement of several chambers, the pattern is more complicated and its interpretation may be difficult. In addition to evaluating the configuration of the margins of the heart itself, one has to observe carefully the location and relative size of the pulmonary trunk and aorta as well as of the pulmonary vasculature. The effect of abnormalities of the thoracic cage has to be taken into account as well. The heart may appear enlarged in the frontal projection if the sagittal diameter of the thoracic cage is decreased. This is the case in the *straight back syndrome* and in *pectus excavatum.*

*Left ventricle:*
- cardiac apex bulges down and left
- positive Hoffman–Rigler sign on lateral view: the posterior border of the left ventricle extends 1.8 cm or more posteriorly to the posterior border of the inferior vena cava at a level 2 cm cephalad to their crossing.

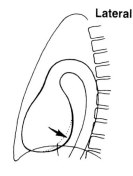
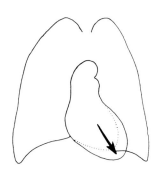

**Lateral**

*Left atrium:*
- esophagus displaced posteriorly
- prominent left auricle
- dense left atrial shadow, double contour on the right
- elevated left main bronchus
- left lower lobe collapse in an extreme case, due to obstructed left lower lobe bronchus

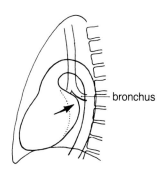
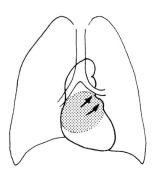

bronchus

*Right ventricle:*
- cardiac enlargement toward left with elevated apex
- filling of retrosternal space
- may displace right atrium toward right
- may displace left ventricle backwards
- 8.4often poorly seen except for pulmonary stenosis, tetralogy of Fallot, etc.

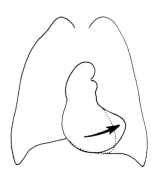

*Right atrium:*
- right heart border beyond ⅓ of the right hemithorax
- may fill the retrosternal space
- rare as a solitary findings

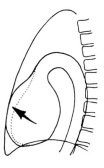
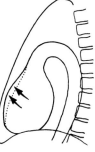
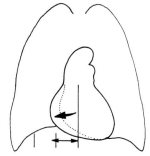

Fig. 1.**4** Typical manifestations of the enlargement of individual cardiac chambers

Evaluation of a suspected congenital heart disease is a difficult task and often it is impossible to name a specific diagnosis without ultrasound examination, catheterization or angiography. A dynamic MRI examination is also diagnostic. When analyzing plain films, the following morphological features should be evaluated in each case:

1 cardiac enlargement – which chambers are enlarged?
2 the size of the aorta- small, wide, narrow, dilated?
3 the vascular pedicle – narrow or wide?
4 right-sided aortic arch?
5 a notch in the aortic arch, resulting in a number 3 appearance?
6 pulmonary vascularity: are the main trunks of the pulmonary artery wide or unusually narrow; is there pulmonary oligemia or hyperemia?
7 the pulmonary artery segment in the left cardiac shadow: large and convex or small and concave.
8 rib notching (Fig. 1.**39**).

The following clinical information is important in evaluating suspected congenital heart disease:

1 is the patient cyanotic or not?
2 Is there right- or left-sided dominance in electrocardiography?
3 Are there typical murmurs?

By using the radiographic and clinical information, it is possible to classify congenital heart diseases of childhood into various groups as presented in Table 1.**1** or often to predict the correct diagnosis, unless multiple defects exist.

In a neonate, only two congenital heart diseases can be diagnosed with great certainty because of their characteristic appearance in chest roentgenogram, namely, *total anomalous pulmonary venous return* (snowman heart) (Fig. 1.**47**) and *pulmonary stenosis with atrial septal defect* (prominent main pulmonary trunk with oligemic lungs). In other cases further clinical information is very helpful in narrowing down the differential diagnostic possibilities. Nowadays ultrasound and Doppler ultrasound examinations have largely replaced plain radiographic analysis of heart.

Based on the time of appearance of cardiac failure and cyanosis, the patients can be divided into the following groups:

1 Cardiac failure manifests early (at birth or during the first week) but there is no cyanosis: *hypoplasia of the left heart; atresia of the aortic* (and *possibly mitral) valve; coarctation of aorta.*
2 Cardiac failure develops later: *ventricular septal defect; patent ductus arteriosus; truncus arteriosus; total anomalous pulmonary venous return (TAPVR).*
3 Cyanosis develops at birth or within a week: *transposition of great vessels; hypoplastic right heart; Ebstein's anomaly; tricuspid atresia; obstructive type of TAPVR.*
4 Cyanosis develops later during childhood: *tetralogy of Fallot; pulmonary stenosis with atrial septal defect.*

Table 1.**3** gives the approximate relative frequency of the congenital heart diseases. In Table 1.**5**, the diseases are grouped according to their dominant, most common or earliest findings. The differential diagnostic groupings in Table 1.**2** may be helpful in narrowing the differential diagnosis in congenital heart diseases in children.

In the adult patient with suspected congenital heart disease, the following features are of particular importance: the position of the diaphragm (high or low); degree of inspiration; calcifications; Kerley B-lines; the appearance of the branches of the pulmonary artery; possible arteriovenous malformations in the lung parenchym anomalous veins across the lung field.

## Evaluation of Blood Flow and Blood Pressure in Lungs

When blood circulation through the lungs is increased, both arteries and veins are full of blood. This occurs in left-to-right shunting (Table 1.**1**) and to a milder degree in hyperkinetic conditions (*hypervolemia, anemia, polycytemia, pregnancy, hyperthyroidism*). A clear oligemia may be a result of a right-to-left shunt or narrow or obliterated pulmonary arterial channels (*narrow pulmonary artery, thromboembolic disease* or*emphysema*). Pulmonary blood flow can increase two to three times before the arterial pressure increases. When the precapillary pressure increases, the peripheral branches of the pulmonary arteries appear narrow, but the central trunks are wide.

An increase in the pulmonary venous pressure causes characteristic changes in the distribution of blood in the lungs. On upright films of an adult untreated patient, such changes relatively accurately reflect the pulmonary venous and left atrial pressure as diagrammatically presented in Fig. 1.**5**. These changes, together with the less sensitive changes in the size and configuration of the heart, are the cornerstone of the radiographic diagnosis of congestive heart failure. The findings in the most common conditions involving left ventricular strain are presented in Table 1.**4**. Although the radiologic evaluation of the pulmonary venous pressure is relatively accurate, the evaluation of venous pressure of the right side is difficult on roentgenograms and is better assessed from the filling of the veins of the patient's neck. Occasionally a prominent azygos vein may be seen (Fig. 1.**6 a**). In conditions such as acute myocardial infarction, even the central venous pressure readings do not reliably reflect the patient's hemodynamic condition.

*Pericardial effusion* mimics generalized cardiomegaly. Although it sometimes may cause a characteristic (bottle-like) configuration of the heart shadow, most of the cases are difficult to diagnose on plain films, and as much as 200 ml of pericardial fluid usually goes undetected in the primary reading. Ultrasound examination CT or MRI are far more sensitive than plain films in detecting pericardial effusion.

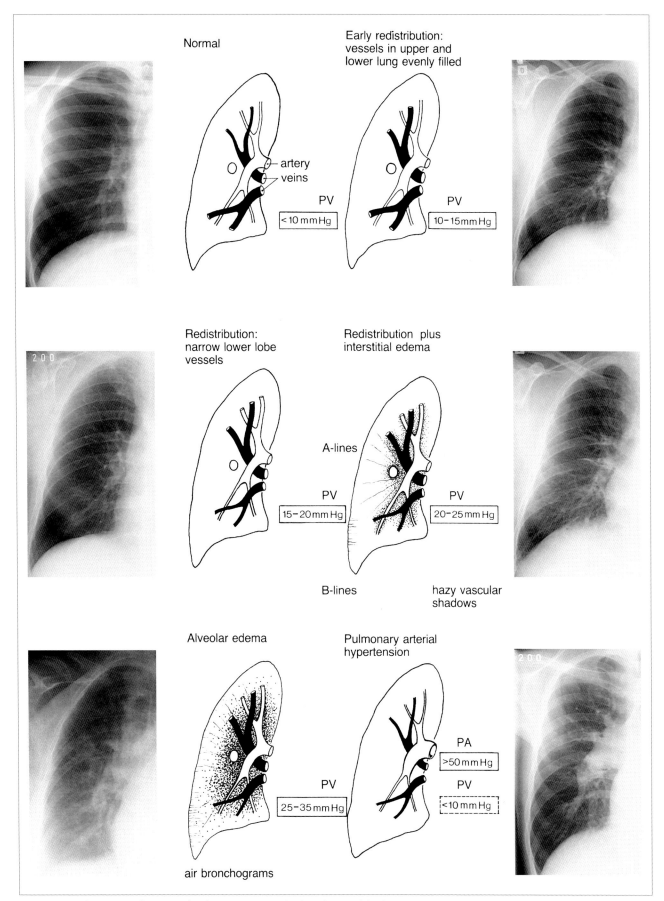

Fig. 1.5   Manifestations of increased pulmonary venous (PV) and arterial (PA) pressure.

**Table 1.5 Predominantly Left Ventricular or Generalized Cardiac Enlargement**

| Disease | Radiographic Findings | Comments |
|---|---|---|
| Athlete's heart (no disease) | Generalized cardiomegaly with left ventricular prominence, no pulmonary vascular changes. | Associated with bradycardia (large stroke volume); secondary to excessive training. |
| Arteriosclerotic heart disease (myocardial ischemia) | Chest roentgenogram is usually unrevealing. Variable degrees of generalized or left ventricular enlargement may occur. | Calcification of the coronary arteries indicates coronary atherosclerosis. |
| Acute myocardial infarction (Figs. 1.6–1.8) | Chest roentgenogram is often unrevealing. Some cardiac dilatation, with variable degrees of pulmonary venous congestion, occurs frequently. Acute pulmonary edema may ensue. | Myocardial aneurysm may develop early in the infarcted muscle or later in the scar. It is seen as a bulge or an unusual prominence in the left ventricular border, which occasionally calcifies. |
| Postmyocardial infarction syndrome (Dressler's syndrome) | Rapid increase in the heart size due to pericardial effusion, always accompanied by either pleural effusion and/or pulmonary infiltrates in the left base or bilaterally. | Can occur a few days or up to two months following an acute infarction. Left-sided or bilateral pleural effusion is the most common finding (80%) and may occur alone. Pericardial effusion is present in 70% and pulmonary infiltrates in 60% of cases. Response to steroid therapy is striking. |

*(continues on page 12)*

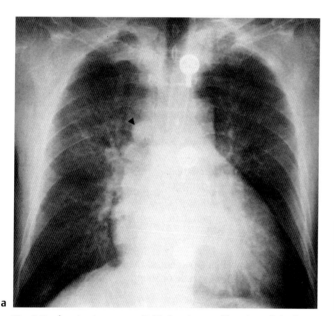
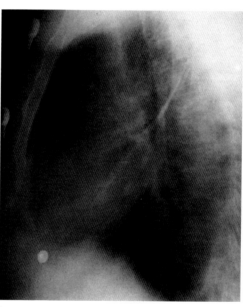

a       b

Fig. 1.**6 a, b** Acute myocardial infarction, **a** dilatation of the heart, pulmonary edema, and congestion of the azygos veins (arrowhead). **b** Lateral view reveals pleural effusion in the pleural fissures.

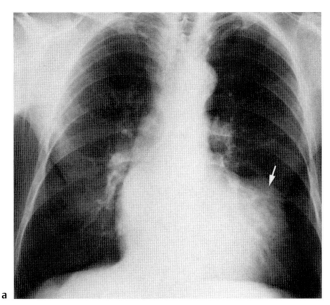
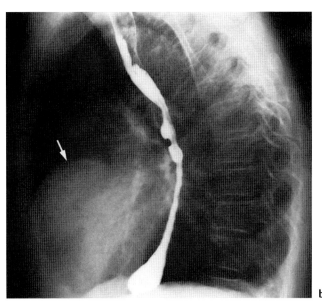

a b

Fig. 1.**7 a, b**    Left ventricular aneurysm after myocardial infarction. A bulge in the cardiac contour is seen in both projections (arrows). Pulmonary vasculature indicates mild venous congestion.

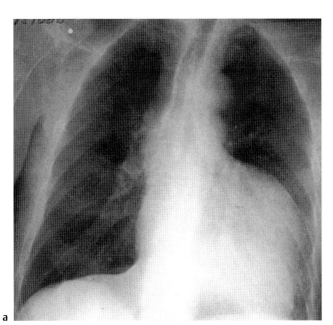
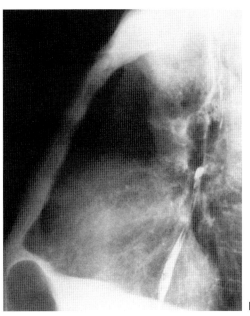

a b

Fig. 1.**8 a, b**    A large left ventricular aneurysm bulges posteriorly, a complication of myocardial infarction. A double density is seen in the AP projection.

**Table 1.5    (Cont.) Predominantly Left Ventricular or Generalized Cardiac Enlargement**

| Disease | Radiographic Findings | Comments |
|---|---|---|
| **Congestive myocardial failure** | | |
| **Left-sided failure (Fig. 1.9)** | Cardiac enlargement, related to the severity of failure and the precongestive heart size. The increase of pulmonary venous pressure can be evaluated as presented in Fig. 1.5). Pleural effusions (bilateral or right-sided). | Pulmonary signs of congestive failure without significant cardiac enlargement. Pericardial calcification is seen in 50%. Often the cardiac configuration resembles that of mitral stenosis.<br>Unilateral left-sided effusion is likely due to causes other than congestive failure. |
| **Right-sided failure (Fig. 1.10)** | Dilatation of the right ventricle and atrium. Widening of the superior vena cava and azygos vein.<br>Liver enlargement. | If right heart failure develops following left heart failure, pulmonary venous congestion from left-sided failure diminishes. |
| **Chronic arterial hypertension (hypertensive heart)** | Left ventricular hypertrophy may produce no radiographic changes or some rounding of the left margin. Left ventricular dilatation causes typical signs of left ventricular enlargement. The aortic knob enlarges concomitantly. Congestive failure may supervene. | Hypertension is most often essential but may be associated *with renal* or *renovascular disease, coarctation of the aorta, adrenal diseases with adrenal hyperfunction, collagen diseases (lupus erythematosus, polyarteritis nodosa),* or *hyperthyroidism.* |
| **Aortic valve insufficiency (Aortic regurgitation) (Fig. 1.11)** | Dilated left ventricle, concave left cardiac border, some dilatation of the ascending aorta and sometimes calcification of the aortic annulus or even the valves. Congestive failure may supervene in advanced cases. Radiographic findings may be subtle although findings in ultrasonography may be obvious. | Insufficiency of the aortic valve can be secondary to:<br>1 primary damage of the valve (e.g., *rheumatoid endocarditis, bacterial endocarditis, congenital valvular deformity, lues, ankylosing spondylitis and Reiter's disease, mucopolysaccharidosis, spontaneous or traumatic rupture of the valve,* or *degenerative phenomena*);<br>2 diseases of the aortic wall or annulus fibrosus (e. g., *cystic medial necrosis, Marfan's syndrome, dissecting aneurysm, lues, arterial hypertension*); or<br>3 congenital malformation of the aortic root (e. g., *aneurysm of the sinus of Valsalva, congenital coronary fistula,* or *high ventricular septal defect with prolapse of the noncoronary cusp*).<br>Congenital aortic insufficiency is usually due to a bicuspid valve.<br>*Acute* aortic insufficiency occurs in *bacterial endocarditis, rupture of the valve* or *dissecting aneurysm.* |

*(continues on page 14)*

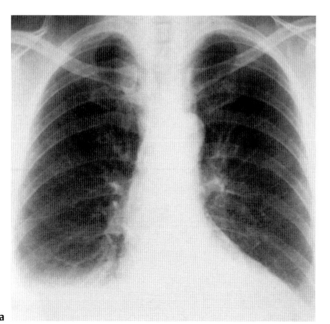
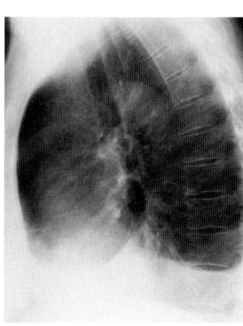

a        b

Fig. 1.**9 a, b**   Chronic left heart failure. There is left ventricular enlargement, pulmonary venous congestion and bilateral pleural Effusion, more on the right side.

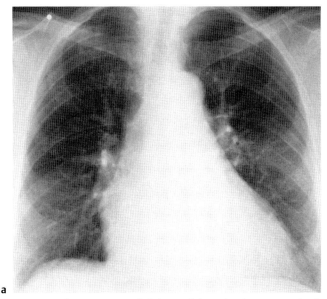
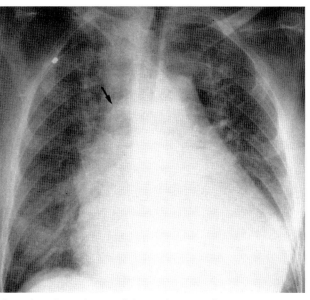

a
b

Fig. 1.**10a, b**   Congestive left heart failure developing into both left- and right-sided failure. **a** Left ventricular enlargement and pulmonary venous congestion. **b** Enlargement of the heart, including the right side, widening of the mediastinum (superior vena cava, and severe pulmonary venous congestion). The azygos vein is also congested (arrow).

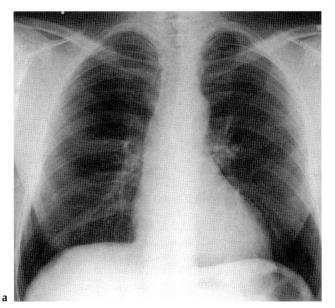
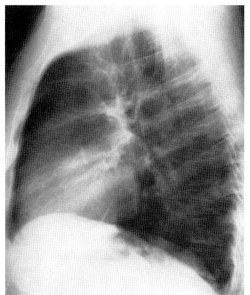

a
b

Fig. 1.**11**   Arteriosclerotic aortic valve insufficiency with mild left ventricular enlargement, no congestive heart failure, and a normal-looking aorta.

## Table 1.5 (Cont.) Predominantly Left Ventricular or Generalized Cardiac Enlargement

| Disease | Radiographic Findings | Comments |
|---|---|---|
| **Combined aortic valve insufficiency and stenosis (Fig. 1.12)** | Dilatation of the left ventricle and ascending aorta is more prominent and left atrium may enlarge. May mimic pure aortic stenosis. | Rheumatoid heart disease usually causes a combination of aortic valve stenosis and insufficiency. |
| **Subvalvular aortic stenosis (idiopathic hypertrophic subaortic stenosis)** | Enlarged left ventricle, often enlarged left atrium. Poststenotic aortic dilatation is absent. | Narrowing of the left ventricular outflow tract by muscular hypertrophy. Essentially ultrasonographic diagnosis. |
| **Supravalvular aortic stenosis** | The heart may be enlarged or normal, the aorta is normal or small. | Congenital fibrous ring or thickening above the sinuses of Valsalva. Frequently associated with idiopathic hypercalcemia of infancy. |
| **Aortic stenosis** | | See Table 1.9 |
| **High-output heart** | Cardiac enlargement, dilatation of the main pulmonary artery, prominent pulmonary vasculature (both arteries and veins). | *Associated conditions:*<br>Pregnancy or athletic (physiological).<br>Severe anemia including sickle-cell anemia, leukemia, or primary polycythemia.<br>Beriberi (vitamin B deficiency). Hypervolemia (fluid overload). Extrapulmonary arteriovenous fistula.<br>Mild forms occur in extreme obesity, thyrotoxicosis, and pyrexia.<br>Advanced Paget's disease is a rare cause of high-output heart. |
| **Myocardiopathy (Figs. 1.13–1.14)** | Diffuse enlargement of the heart, predominantly of the left ventricle. The aorta appears small as compared with the size of the heart. Pulmonary venous congestion may develop. Moderate left atrial enlargement and fullness of the main pulmonary artery occurs. Superimposed pericardial effusion may further enlarge the cardiac shadow. | The many causes of myocardiopathy may be classified into five groups:<br>1 Idiopathic, unassociated with extracardiac disease: *non-specific myocardosis; endocardial fibroelastosis (neonate or child); postpartum cardiopathy.*<br>2 Infectious: *Coxsackie B and other viral infections; Chagas' disease (South American trypanosomiasis) ; rheumatic, septic, diphtheric, toxoplasmic.*<br>3 Infiltrative: *amyloidosis (especially primary), generalized glycogen storage disease (Pompe's disease, infant); leukemia.*<br>4 Endocrine: *hypothyroidism; acromegaly; Cushing's disease; thyrotoxicosis.*<br>5 Miscellaneous causes: *ischemic; uremia; collagen diseases; nutritional deficiency (beriberi, alcoholism, potassium or magnesium depletion); toxicity (drugs, chemicals, cobalt); sarcoidosis; neuromuscular dystrophy.*<br>A combination of cardiac enlargement and normal pulmonary vasculature is usually due to one of the following four entities:<br>1 myocardiopathy; 2 aortic stenosis; 3 aortic coarctation, or 4 athlete's heart. |

*(continues on page 16)*

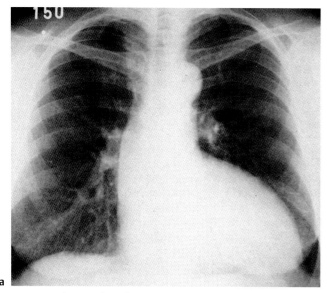

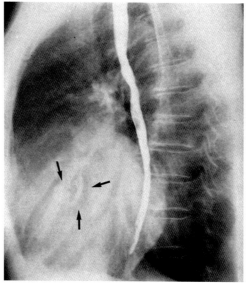

a

b

Fig. 1.**12 a, b**   Combined aortic valve stenosis and insufficiency of rheumatic origin. Extensive enlargement of the left ventricle and dilated ascending aorta. Aortic valve calcification is demonstrated (arrows)

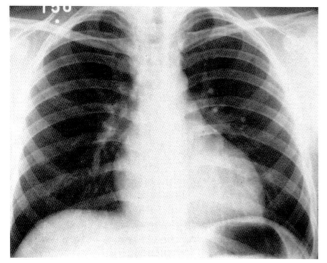

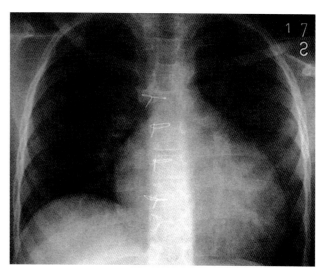

Fig. 1.**13**   Uremic myocardiopathy. Left ventricular enlargement without congestive failure. The aorta is relatively small.

Fig. 1.**14**   Diabetic cardiomyopathy in a child aged 10,The heart is large, and left ventricles is very prominent. Pulmonary vasculature is normal.

## Table 1.5 (Cont.) Predominantly Left Ventricular or Generalized Cardiac Enlargement

| Disease | Radiographic Findings | Comments |
|---|---|---|
| **Mitral insufficiency** **Coarctation of aorta** **Patent ductus arteriosus** **Ventricular septal defect** | Left ventricular enlargement is a feature in these conditions as well as in a number of rare congenital heart diseases. | Since other characteristics are more useful for differential diagnosis they will be discussed elsewhere. |
| **Pericardial defect** **(Fig. 1.15)** | 1 Displacement of the heart to left without displacement of trachea. 2 Unusual configuration of the left heart border (bulging aortic, pulmonary arterial and left ventricular segments). 3 Bulging through a partial defect may mimic left ventricular aneurysm, but shows no paradoxal pulsations. | Either total (in 3/4) or partial absence of pericardium, usually on the left side, which usually is symptomless and discovered incidentally. Displacement of the heart may simulate left ventricular enlargement. A deep notch between the aorta and pulmonary artery is characteristic. |
| **Acute glomerulonephritis in children** | Generalized cardiomegaly Pleural effusions Pulmonary interstitial or alveolar edema | Cardiac dilatation occurs in over 50% of acute cases in children. The mechanism is unknown. The radiographic changes subside together with healing of the underlying disease. |
| **Pericardial effusion** **(Fig. 1.16, Fig. 1.17)** | Enlarged cardiac shadow mimics generalized cardiomegaly. Large effusions tend to obliterate normal cardiac markings. There is less posterior displacement of the barium-filled esophagus in the lateral view than could be expected from the apparent heart size. Rapid changes occur in the cardiac silhouette in consecutive films, in the absence of pulmonary vascular enlargement. Postural alterations change cardiac contours. The pulmonary vasculature is decreased and the superior vena cava may be prominent if tamponade of the right atrial inflow occurs. | Common causes of pericardial effusion are: *Pericarditis* (especially Coxsackie virus, but also in other infections) *Congestive heart failure* *Collagen diseases (LED)* *Cardiac surgery or trauma* *Renal failure* *Postmyocardial infarction syndrome* *Tumor invasion* (from lung or mediastinal lymphoma) or metastases (from lung, breast, or melanoma) *Radiation therapy* *Still's disease* |
| **Transposition of great vessels** **(Fig. 1.18)** | "Egg-on-side" cardiomegaly that appears during the first week after birth together with congestive heart failure. Concave pulmonary artery segment, although vascularity in the lungs is increased unless transposition is associated with pulmonary stenosis, the latter occurs in 15%. Narrow vascular pedicle in frontal projection (aorta and pulmonary artery are superimposed), seen in 50%. | A rare anomaly, but the most frequent form of congenital heart disease associated with cyanosis present since birth. Due to lack of spiralization of the spiral septum, the aorta remains anterior and originates from the right ventricle. The pulmonary artery is behind the aorta and originates from the left ventricle. Pulmonary and systemic circulation are connected through a defect in the atrial and/or ventricular septum or through a patent ductus arteriosus. |
| **Tricuspid atresia** | | See Table 1.7 |
| **Anomalous left coronary artery** | Radiographic changes are identical to other myocardiopathies such as endocardial fibroelastosis (see under myocardiopathy in this Table, above). | Left coronary artery originating from the pulmonary artery is the most common significant anomaly of the coronary circulation. |

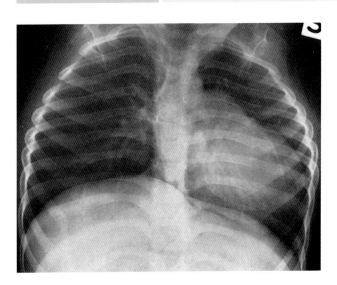

Fig. 1.**15** Pericardial defect, age 5. The heart (not mediastinum) is displaced to the left. The aortic, pulmonary, and left ventricular segments are sharply bulging, a characteristic pattern.

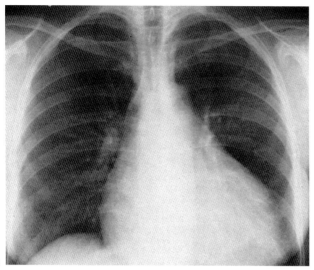
a

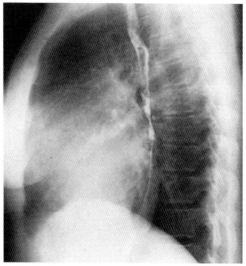
b

Fig. 1.**16 a, b**    Pericardial effusion. The cardiac shadow is large, but the esophagus in the lateral view is not proportionally displaced posteriorly.

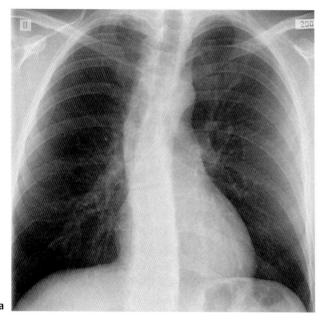
a

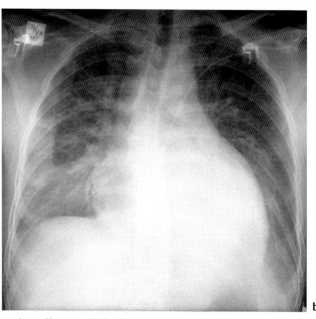
b

Fig. 1.**17 a, b**    Still's disease. Fig. 1.**17 a** was taken one month before than Fig. 1.**17 b**. Massive increase in heart size is due to peri- cardiac effusion which also caused emerging heart tamponade and pulmonary constriction.

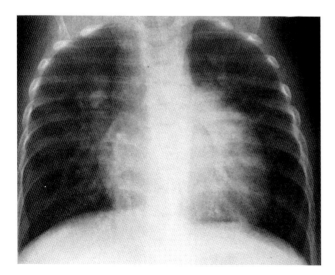

Fig. 1.**18**    Transposition of great vessels. "Egg-on-side" cardiomegaly and a concave pulmonary segment associated with increased vascularity of lungs. Narrow vascular pedicle.

## Table 1.6 Predominantly Left Atrial Enlargement

| Disease | Radiographic Findings | Comments |
|---|---|---|
| **Mitral stenosis (acquired or congenital) (Figs. 1.19–20)** | 1. Left atrial enlargement<br>2. Possible calcification of the mitral valve, not to be confused with the heavy calcification of the mitral anulus<br>3. Pulmonary venous congestion<br>4. Prominent main pulmonary artery segment, enlarged hilar vessels<br>5. A small aortic knob<br>6. Right ventricular enlargement, normal-sized left ventricle<br>7. Dilatation of the central pulmonary arteries and narrowing of peripheral arteries (pulmonary arterial hypertension)<br>8. Pulmonary parenchymal changes due to hemosiderosis (granular opacities) (Fig. 5.**47**, p. 117), multiple up to 8 mm ossifications, or pulmonary fibrosis (pulmonary infarctions) | Obstruction of flow from the left atrium into the left ventricle during diastole, resulting in increased pressure and enlargement of the left atrium. The increased pressure is transmitted to the pulmonary veins and eventually to the pulmonary arteries and the right heart. The usual cause is a *rheumatic* valvular lesion. *Congenital mitral stenosis* can be identical to the rheumatic one (short chordae tendineae, fibrotic valves and fused commissures). A rare congenital form of mitral stenosis is the *parachute deformity* (all chordae tendineae originate from a single papillary muscle). The latter is associated with other anomalies. In the early phase, congenital mitral stenosis and a left-to-right shunt may appear similar but in mitral stenosis the vascular shadows are hazier due to venous and lymphatic congestion. Enlarged confluence of right pulmonary veins may mimic left atrial enlargement or tumor. |

*(continues on page 20)*

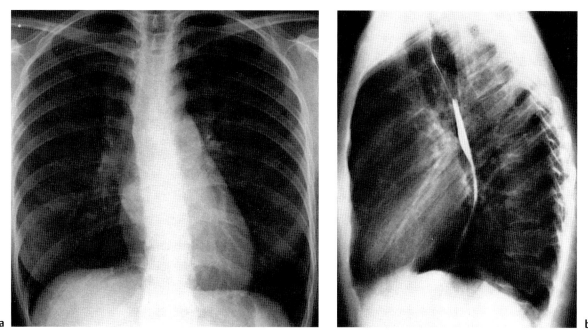

Fig. 1.**19 a, b**   Mitral stenosis, early. The left atrium is enlarged and seen as a double density in the PA projection. It displaces the esophagus posteriorly. Pulmonary vasculature is unremarkable.

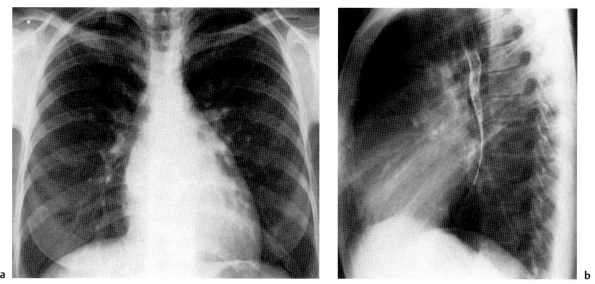

Fig. 1.**20 a, b**   Mitral stenosis. Enlarged left atrium, right ventricle, and main pulmonary artery segment, pulmonary venous congestion and a small aortic knob.

**Table 1.6 (Cont.) Predominantly Left Atrial Enlargement**

| Disease | Radiographic Findings | Comments |
|---|---|---|
| **Mitral insufficiency (mitral regurgitation) (Figs. 1.21–24)** | 1 Enlarged, sometimes enormous left atrium<br>2 Enlarged left ventricle<br>3 Small or normal aortic knob<br>4 Normal pulmonary vasculature, sometimes venous congestion and prominent pulmonary artery are present. | Most commonly caused by *rheumatic valvulitis*, but may also be caused by functional dilatation of the mitral ring secondary to other cardiac diseases (*congestive heart failure, acute rheumatic fever, aortic valve disease, coarctation of aorta*), or from *papillary muscle dysfunction*. Regurgitation of blood during ventricular systole leads to overfilling and dilatation of the left atrium and dilatation of the left ventricle.<br>In most cases both valvular conditions (stenosis and insufficiency) coexist, giving a mixed pattern, Mitral disease is often associated with aortic disease or tricuspid disease or both, which results in a complicated radiographic pattern. |
| **Myxoma of the left atrium** | The heart may have a configuration of mitral stenosis. Calcification of the tumor is rare, but helpful in differential diagnosis if present. | Myxoma is the most common tumor of the heart, which usually occurs in the left atrium. |
| **Patent ductus arteriosus**<br>**ventricular septal defect**<br>**myocardiopathy**<br>**congenital coronary fistula**<br>**triogy of Fallot**<br>**tricuspid atresia** | Left atrial enlargement may be a significant feature in these conditions. | Other radiographic changes are more diagnostic and these entities are presented elsewhere in this Chapter. |

*(continues on page 22)*

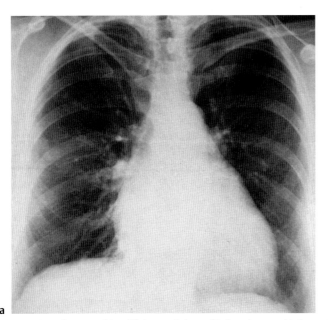 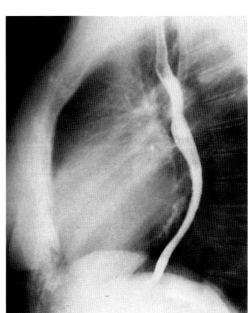

a        b

Fig. 1.**21 a, b** Mitral insufficiency. Enlarged left atrium and left ventricle, small aortic knob. Normal pulmonary vasculature.

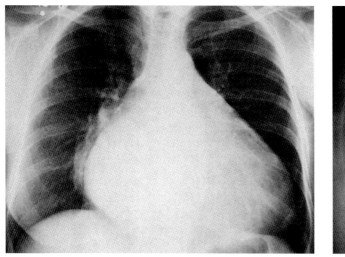
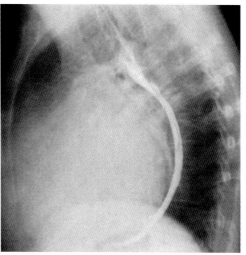

Fig. 1.**22 a, b**    Mitral insufficiency. Enormous left atrium, dilatation of the left ventricle and generalized cardiomegaly with small aortic knob.

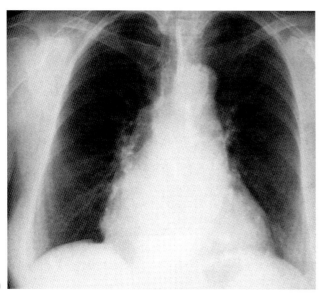
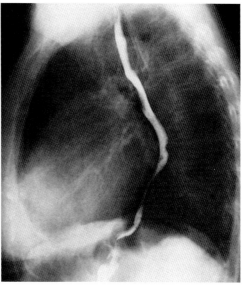

Fig. 1.**23 a, b**    Combined mitral stenosis and insufficiency. Enlargement of left atrium and both ventricles. Pulmonary venous congestion.

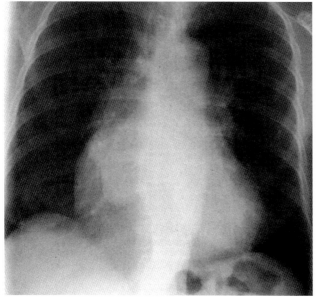
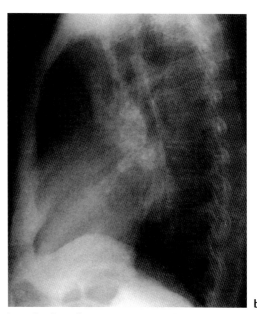

Fig. 1.**24 a, b**    Confluence of right pulmonary veins mimicking enlarged left atrium. The patient has aortic and mitral insufficiency and pulmonary venous congestion. The bulge caused by an en- larged right pulmonary venous confluence is more localized than an enlargement of the left atrium and may mimic a tumor, **a** Oblique and **b** lateral views.

**Table 1.6  (Cont.) Predominantly Left Atrial Enlargement**

| Disease | Radiographic Findings | Comments |
|---|---|---|
| **Constrictive pericarditis (Fig. 1.25)** | Pulmonary venous congestion without cardiac enlargement. Left atrium is usually prominent. Calcification of the pericardium may be seen. The pattern mimics mitral stenosis. | Lack of calcification does not exclude constrictive pericarditis. Conversely, calcified pericardium is associated with constrictive pericarditis only in about 50% of cases. |
| **Single ventricle (cor triloculare biatriatum) (Fig. 1.26)** | Plain film findings are not diagnostic. Left atrium is often enlarged and pulmonary vasculature increased, sometimes suggestive of ventricular septal defect. | A single functional ventricle usually associated with other anomalies, most often pulmonary artery stenosis. |

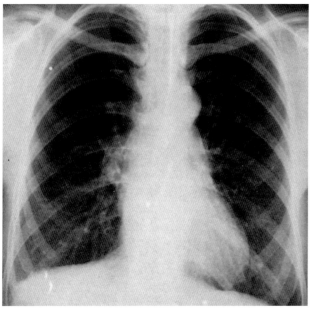
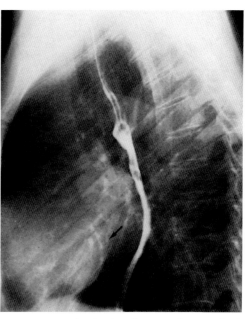

a  b

Fig. 1.**25 a, b**  Constrictive pericarditis. Enlarged left atrium displaces barium-filled esophagus in the lateral view. Pulmonary venous congestion in the absence of generalized cardiornegaly mimics mitral stenosis. Pericardial calcification (arrow).

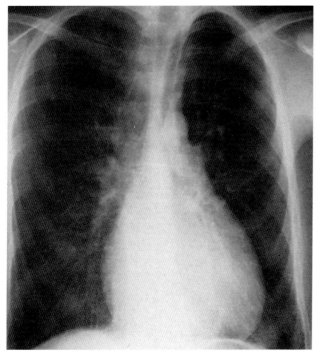
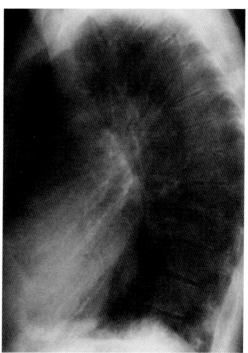

a  b

Fig. 1.**26 a, b**  Single ventricle. Mild cardiomegaly, prominent left atrium, small aorta, and increased pulmonary vascularity.

## Table 1.7    Predominantly Right Ventricular Enlargement

| Disease | Radiographic Findings | Comments |
|---|---|---|
| **Tetralogy of Fallot** (Figs. 1.27–28) | Changes depend on the degree of pulmonary stenosis and the size of the septal defect. <br>1 Right ventricular enlargement causes elevation of the cardiac apex but heart is not particularly big. <br>2 Pulmonary blood vessels are either oligemic or normal-looking. <br>3 The main pulmonary artery segment is concave or small. <br>4 The size of the aorta is normal or enlarged. Right-sided aortic arch is present in 25%. <br>5 Short straight lines in lungs represent enlarged bronchial arteries. | The most common cyanotic congenital heart disease. Primary changes are infundibular pulmonary stenosis and a high ventricular septal defect. Overriding of the aorta and right ventricular hypertrophy are secondary structural defects. Mixing of venous blood with arterial blood leads to cyanosis after closure of ductus arteriosus. The smaller the pulmonary artery, the bigger the aorta. A typical radiographic appearance is present only in one-third of cases. If pulmonary stenosis is minimal, the clinical picture is as in ventricular septal defect. If foramen ovale persists, the condition is called *pentalogy of Fallot*. |

*(continues on page 24)*

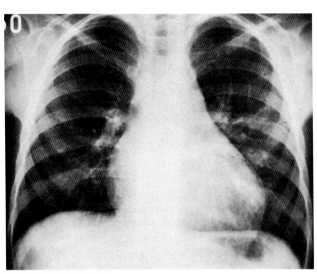 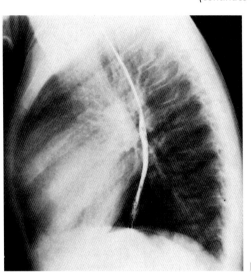

a          b

Fig. 1.**27 a, b**    Tetralogy of Fallot in a child. The right ventricle is enlarged but the main pulmonary segment is concave, and the pulmonary blood vessels normal-looking or slightly oligemic.

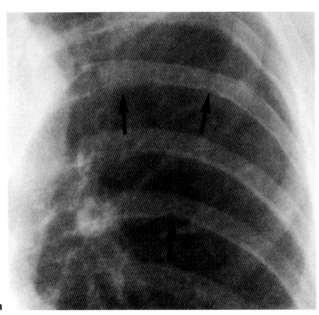 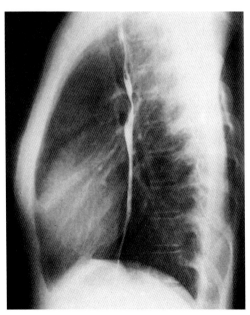

a          b

Fig. 1.**28 a, b**    Tetralogy of Fallot after Blalock operation, age 17, Relatively small heart but apex still elevated and pulmonary artery segment very small. Rib notching post-Blalockoperation (arrows).

## Table 1.7 (Cont.) Predominantly Right Ventricular Enlargement

| Disease | Radiographic Findings | Comments |
|---|---|---|
| **Tricuspid atresia (mimics right ventricular enlargement) (Fig. 1.29)** | "Pure" tricuspidal atresia<br>1 Normal or slightly enlarged heart size.<br>2 The left heart border is rounded and elevated, simulating right ventricular enlargement.<br>3 Concave main pulmonary artery segment.<br>4 Pulmonary oligemia with eventual reticular densities representing bronchial arteries.<br>5 Right-sided aortic arch (in 20%).<br>6 Left atrial enlargement (in 50%). | Congenital obliteration of the tricuspid valve that results in early cyanosis. Blood that should flow into the right ventricle is deviated through an atrial septal defect or foramen ovale into the left atrium and into the enlarged left ventricle. The roentgenographic appearance may mimic tetralogy of Fallot but electrocardiography shows left axis deviation (right axis deviation in Pallet's tetralogy). Usually associated with pulmonary artery obstruction (infundibular stenosis or pulmonary valvular atresia). |
| | If associated with transposition of great vessels (in more than 1/4 of cases) the appearance is different:<br>1 The aorta is small.<br>2 Pulmonary vasculature is increased.<br>3 The abnormally located right auricular appendage bulges in the left upper cardiac border. | Tricuspid atresia with transposition of great vessels may be present with or without pulmonary arterial obstruction. |
| **Truncus arteriosus (common aorticopulmonary trunk) (Fig. 1.30)** | 1 Right ventricular enlargement in a slightly enlarged heart<br>2 Absence of the usual main pulmonary artery (concave pulmonary artery segment)<br>3 Hypervascular lungs (types I-III). If pulmonary arteries are hypoplastic, lungs are hypovascular (type IV).<br>4 Right-sided aortic arch in one-fourth of cases | A usually fatal failure of the development of the spiral septum. Several forms of the takeoff of pulmonary arteries from the common trunk, including absence of pulmonary arteries (type IV), which results in a radiographic picture similar to the tetralogy of Fallot. |
| **Pseudotruncus arteriosus** | 1 Large right ventricle<br>2 Concave main pulmonary artery segment<br>3 Pulmonary oligemia (bronchial arteries may be seen)<br>4 Right-sided aortic arch<br>The plain film appearance of pseudotruncus is identical to tetralogy of Fallot. | The term pseudotruncus arteriosus is used to designate atresia of the pulmonary valve or the main pulmonary trunk, associated with a ventricular septal defect. There is an intracardiac right-to-left shunt (VSD) and a left-to-right shunt at patent ductus arteriosus. |
| **Chronic left heart failure (myocardiopathy, mitral insufficiency) Mitral stenosis** | Right ventricular enlargement occurs often in these conditions secondary to pulmonary arterial hypertension. | See Tables 1.5 and 1.6 |
| **Cor pulmonale Left-to-right shunt Pulmonary stenosis** | Increased flow or pressure causes enlargement of the right ventricle in these conditions. | Enlargement of the main pulmonary artery segment is a more sensitive sign and easier to appreciate. Hence, these conditions are discussed under the enlargement of pulmonary artery segment (Table 1.10). |

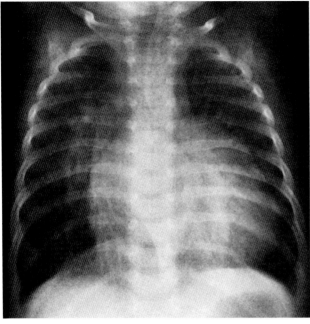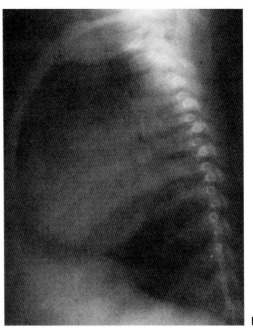

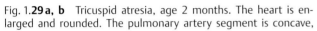

Fig. 1.**29 a, b**   Tricuspid atresia, age 2 months. The heart is enlarged and rounded. The pulmonary artery segment is concave, and the left atrium is enlarged. The reticular vascular pattern represents enlarged bronchial arteries.

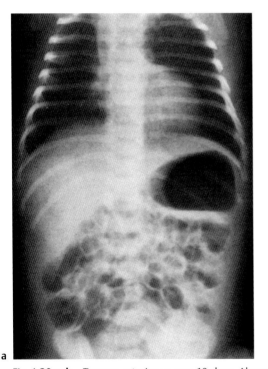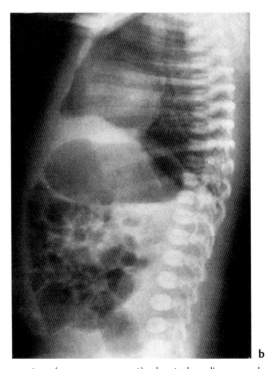

Fig. 1.**30 a, b**   Truncus arteriosus, age 10 days, Absence of pulmonary artery (concave segment), elevated cardiac apex, hypovascular lungs, and right-sided aortic arch.

**Table 1.8 Right Atrial Enlargement or Prominent Right Heart Border**

| Disease | Radiographic Findings | Comments |
|---|---|---|
| Pericardial cyst or lipoma (Figs. 1.31–32) | A localized bulge usually at the cardiophrenic angle; no cardiovascular abnormality. | Fat or fluid content can be demonstrated with CT |
| Hypoplasia of the lung and/or pulmonary artery (Fig. 1.33) | Displacement of the normal-sized heart shadow towards right. Vessels of the lung may be abnormally small (arterial hypo-plasia). The diaphragm may be elevated, the hemithorax smaller, and an abnormal vein (scimitar syndrome) may be seen across the tower lung field (pulmonary hypo-plasia). | |
| Tricuspid stenosis and insufficiency | 1  Rounding of the right cardiac border<br>2  Prominent superior vena cava<br>3  Elevated right hemidiaphragm due to enlarged liver. | Usually a rheumatic lesion of the tricuspid valve. Tricuspid stenosis and insufficiency produce identical roentgenographic findings. The condition is almost always associated with mitral and/or aortic valvular diseases that are responsible for overall cardiac enlargement. The rare solitary tricuspid stenosis may occur in *carcinoid syndrome, lupus erythematosus,* or *endomyocardial fibrosis*. |

*(continues on page 28)*

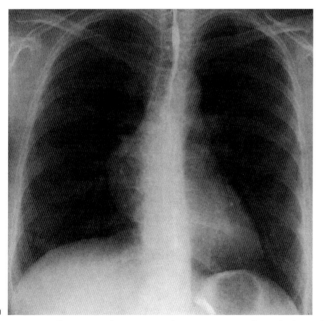 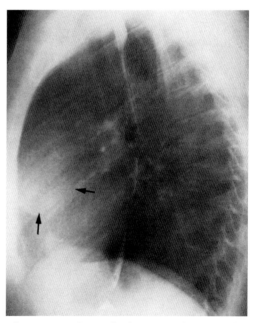

a                                                                                                                   b

Fig. 1.**31 a, b**  Pericardial cyst. A soft-tissue mass in the right heart border mimics right atrial enlargement, but in the lateral view **b** it is seen to be more anterior than the right atrium (arrows).

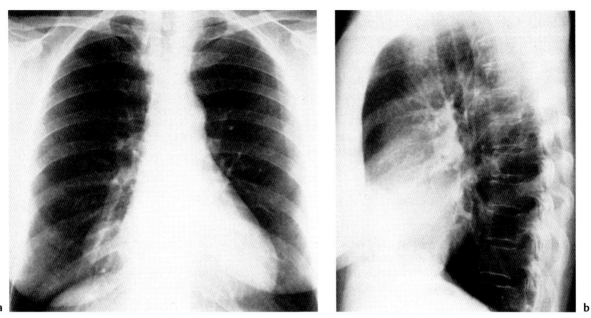

Fig. 1.**32 a, b**   Pericardial lipoma. A low-density mass in the right anterior cardiophrenic angle.

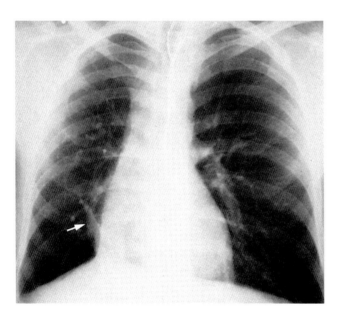

Fig. 1.**33**   Hypoplasia of the right lung with partial anomalous venous return. The mediastinum and right heart border are displaced to the right. The heart size is normal. Anomalous vein drawing into the inferior vena cava (scimitar sign) is seen in the right lower lung field (arrow).

## Table 1.9 (Cont.) Prominent or Malpositioned Ascending Aorta and/or Aortic Arch

| Disease | Radiographic Findings | Comments |
|---|---|---|
| **Aortic valvular stenosis (congenital or acquired) (Fig. 1.39)** | 1  There is little or no enlargement of the heart but the left lower border may present convex bulging.<br>2  Poststenotic dilatation of the ascending aorta while the aortic knob is normal or small.<br>3  Calcifications of the diseased aortic valve increase with age, but may be undetected on high kVp films.<br>4  Dilatation of the left ventricle is a late finding and often followed by congestive failure. | Congenital valvular stenosis is usually associated with bicuspic valves. Radiographic changes are similar to acquired stenosis.<br>Acquired aortic stenosis usually develops on a rheumatic basis and it is often associated with other valvular, especially mitral, involvement. Aortic stenosis may also develop on atherosclerotic basis, but it is usually a combination of stenosis and insufficiency (see Table 1.5). |
| **Aortic insufficiency** | See Table 1.5 | |
| **Coarctation of the aorta (Figs. 1.40–42)** | 1  Dilated or prominent ascending aorta.<br>2  The narrowed segment appears as a notch in the contour of the descending aorta just below the knob.<br>3  Dilated left subclavian artery often produces a bulge above the aortic knob.<br>4  Poststenotic dilatation immediately below the narrowed segment may produce a figure "3" appearance of the descending aorta.<br>5  Dilatation of the internal mammary arteries may be visualized on the lateral film as a soft-tissue density.<br>6  Cardiac enlargement is rarely marked; it usually involves the left ventricle. | Notching of the inferior margins of the ribs (3 to 9) is the most common diagnostic finding in patients over 6 years. |
| **Congenital pseudo-coarctation of the aorta** | Two bulges in the region of the aortic knob, mimicking coarctation, in the absence of other findings typical of coarctation. | Buckling or kinking of the aortic arch in the region of ligamentum arteriosum without obstruction or other hemodynamic abnormality. Asymptomatic if no other abnormalities exist. |

(continues on page 34)

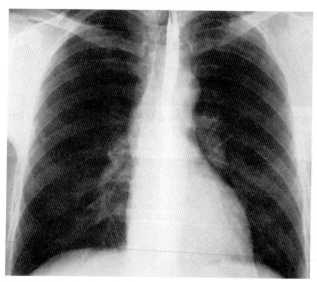
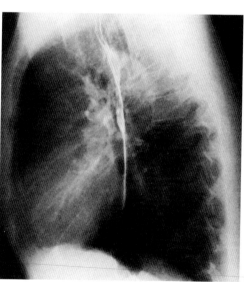

a      b

Fig. 1.**39 a, b**  Aortic valvular stenosis of rheumatic origin, age 32. The heart size is normal but the ascending aorta is too wide in the PA projection, considering the patient's age,

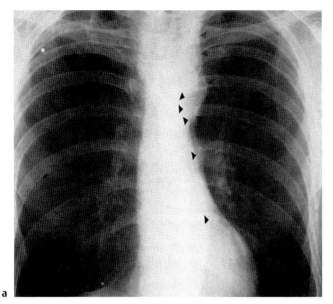
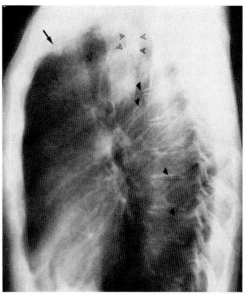

a                                                                b

Fig. 1.**40 a, b**   Coarctation of the aorta, age 59. The aortic knob (^^) is prominent. The narrowing of proximal descending aorta is demonstrated on plain films (^^). Dilated left subclavian artery (A A) and rib notching (–) are characteristic. There is no continuity of   aortic outline between the precoarctation and postcoarctation segments in the posteroanterior view. Dilated internal mammary artery (arrow) is seen behind the manubrium on the lateral film.

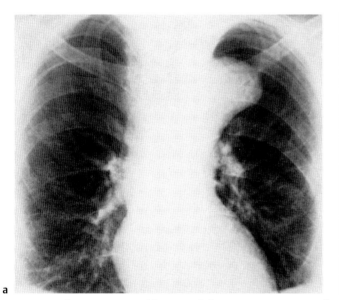
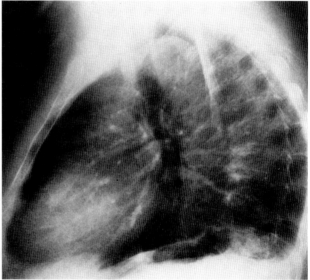

a                                                                b

Fig. 1.**41 a, b**   Poststenotic dilatation of the aorta in a patient with coarctation of aorta and Turner's syndrome(age 43). Fusion of the manubriosternal joint and pectus carinatum are also seen.

Fig. 1.**42**   Coarctation of aorta, postsurgical. The prosthetic segment is seen as a wide loop, which, however, has a normal diameter (arrows).

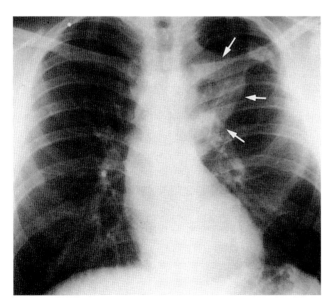

**Table 1.9   (Cont.) Prominent or Malpositioned Ascending Aorta and/or Aortic Arch**

| Disease | Radiographic Findings | Comments |
|---|---|---|
| **Tricuspid atresia without transposition of great vessels and Truncus arteriosus** | Aortic enlargement is a feature of these rare congenital disorders. | See Table 1.7 |
| **Aortic arch malformations (Fig. 1.43)** | Several types occur:<br>1  Right-sided aortic arch with mirror branching of the major arteries.<br>2  Right-sided aortic arch with an aberrant left subclavian artery and persistent left ligamentum arteriosum.<br>3  Anomalous right subclavian artery.<br>4  Double aortic arch (left, right, and posterior indentation of the esophagus) | Anomalous right subclavian artery is the most frequent anomaly. *Indentation of the posterior esophagus* occurs in all but the right-sided arch with mirror branches. In the latter anomaly the aorta is *anterior to esophagus* and trachea. It is almost always associated with cyanotic congenital heart disease (tetralogy of Fallot, truncus arteriosus, transposition of great vessels). |
| **Corrected transposition of great vessels** | Reversed positions of the great vessels and reversed functions of the ventricles.<br>A smooth bulge of the upper left cardiac border is caused by the left-sided ascending aorta. | Uncomplicated corrected transposition is very rare. Associated defects include ventricular septal defect, a single ventricle or pulmonary stenosis. They modify the radiographic appearance. |

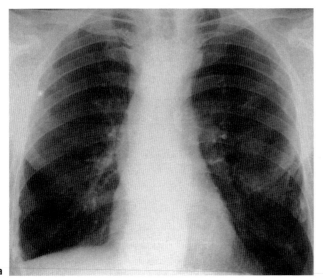
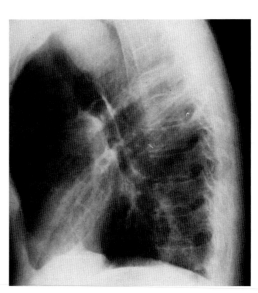

a         b

Fig. 1.**43 a, b**   Right-sided aortic arch. The aorta passes behind the esophagus and is seen as a round mass in the upper mediastinum. Hence, there is no associated congenital heart anomaly. Extensive pleural calcifications (asbestosis), an incidental finding.

## Table 1.10  Dilatation of the Main Pulmonary Artery Segment

| Disease | Radiographic Findings | Comments |
|---|---|---|
| "Idiopathic" (No disease) | Convexity or moderate prominence of the pulmonary artery segment without abnormality. | Physiologic feature in young persons that may persist. Cardiac rotation in pectus excavatum causes a relative prominence of the pulmonary artery segment. In lordotic view and oblique projections the pulmonary artery segment appears prominent. |
| Pregnancy High output heart Congestive heart failure | Moderately enlarged pulmonary artery segment due to increased flow or increased blood volume in pulmonary circulation. | See Table 1.5 |
| Cor pulmonale and Pulmonary arterial hypertension (Fig. 1.44) | 1  Fullness and increased convexity of the main pulmonary artery segment.<br>2  Prominence of the main branches of the pulmonary artery.<br>3  Abrupt decrease of the caliber of the peripheral pulmonary arterial branches may be present, indicating pulmonary hypertension.<br>4  Normal heart size, later right ventricular enlargement.<br>5  If right heart failure supervenes, further cardiac dilatation and distention of the superior vena cava appears, together with eventual pleural fluid. | Cor pulmonale may develop secondary to a variety of conditions, easily overlooked in chest X-rays<br>1  Diffuse lung disease: *chronic obstructive emphysema; interstitial fibrosis* of various causes.<br>2  Diffuse pulmonary arterial diseases: *pulmonary thromboembolism*; (e.g., recurrent emboli, sickle cell anemia); *arteritis* (e.g., polyarteritis nodosa, Wegener's granulomatosis, schistosomiasis); *primary pulmonary hypertension*.<br>3  Chronic heart disease: *left ventricular failure; mitral valve disease; left-to-right shunt*.<br>4  Extrapulmonary causes of hypoventilation (*kyphoscoliosis, obesity, neuromuscular disorders, ankylosing spondylitis*). |
| Pulmonary embolism or thrombosis | Fullness of the main pulmonary artery segment with or without dilatation of the right ventricle is occasionally present in pulmonary embolism or infarction. In most cases the heart appears normal. | In serial films, changes in the main pulmonary artery segment are more frequently observable. |

*(continues on page 36)*

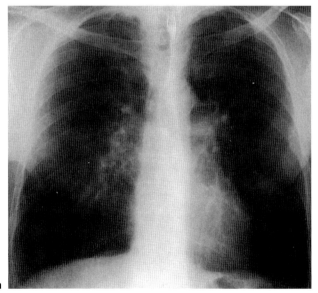
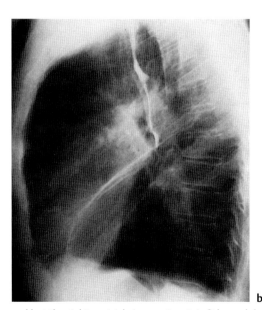

a      b

Fig. 1.**44 a, b**  Cor pulmonale. Wide pulmonary artery segment and main branches. Narrow peripheral pulmonary arteries. Severe chronic obstructive emphysema. The heartsize is otherwise normal but the right ventricle is prominent. Left lower lobe atelectasis is also seen.

## Table 1.10 (Cont.) Dilatation of the Main Pulmonary Artery Segment

| Disease | Radiographic Findings | Comments |
| --- | --- | --- |
| **Atrial septal defect (Fig. 1.45)** | The size of the defect will determine the amount of blood shunted into the pulmonary circulation.<br>1 Enlargement of the main pulmonary artery segment and pulmonary arterial branches.<br>2 Dilatation of the right ventricle and the right atrium.<br>3 The aortic knob is relatively small.<br>4 The left atrium and left ventricle are normal. | The most common defect type is the so called ostium secundum near the foramen ovale. The less common ostium primum defect is just above the mitral valve and may be associated with abnormal mitral and tricuspid valves and a ventricular septal defect (*atrioventricularis communis, endocardial cushion defect*). This defect is most frequently found in association with *Down's syndrome* (mongolism). A defect above the foramen ovale is rare, but often associated with right-sided *anomalous-pulmonary venous return*. Abrupt narrowing of the peripheral arteries and wide central arteries including almost aneurysmatic dilatation of the main pulmonary artery is characteristic of *pulmonary hypertension* (*Eisenmenger's physiology*), that may even reverse the shunt. |
| **Ventricular septal defect (Fig. 1.46)** | 1 Prominent main pulmonary artery segment.<br>2 Increased pulmonary vascularity.<br>3 Enlarged left atrium and left ventricle.<br>4 Small aortic knob.<br>5 The right ventricle may be enlarged.<br>The larger the shunt, the larger the left atrium and left ventricle and the smaller the aortic knob. | The most common congenital heart disease. The size and location of the defect determine its hemodynamic effect. A low muscular defect is usually small and rarely has clinical significance. A high ventricular septal defect near the aortic valve results both anatomically and functionally in an overriding aorta. Increased flow into the right ventricle in such a situation causes right ventricular enlargement and enlargement of the pulmonary artery. If pulmonary hypertension develops, right ventricular enlargement increases but the left ventricle may appear smaller. A defect high in the ventricular septum can cause prolapse of the non-coronary cusp with resultant aortic insufficiency and dilatation of the ascending aorta. |

*(continues on page 38)*

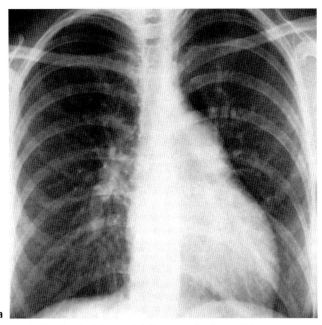
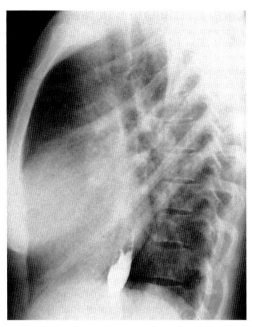

a
b

Fig. 1.**45 a, b**   Atrial septal defact, age 24. Large Pulmonary artery segment and pulmonary arterial branches. Dilated right Ventricle is seen as prominence of the anterior border of the heart.

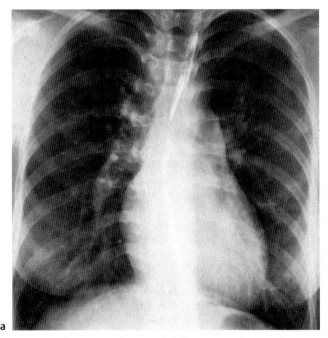
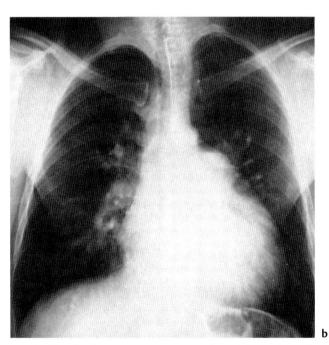

a
b

Fig. 1.**46 a, b**   Ventricular septal defect. **a** Prominent pulmonary artery segment, increased pulmonary vasculature, small aorta,and minimal left ventricular enlargement. Age 20. **b** Another patient, grossly dilated pulmonary artery segment, large left ventricle,pulmonary arterial hypertension (wide but rapidly tapering pulmonary arteries).

### Table 1.10 (Cont.) Dilatation of the Main Pulmonary Artery Segment

| Disease | Radiographic Findings | Comments |
|---|---|---|
| **Patent ductus arterio-sus (Fig. 1.47)** | Radiographic changes depend on the age and volume of shunted blood:<br>1 The main pulmonary artery segment and the central pulmonary arteries are enlarged. Often the right hilar shadow is larger than the left.<br>2 The pulmonary vascularity is increased.<br>3 The left atrium and left ventricle are enlarged and produce moderate cardiomegaly.<br>4 Aorta proximal to the shunt may enlarge. A convex bulge below the aortic knob represents the origin of the ductus. This "infundibulum sign" is present in one-third of patients. | If the ductus arteriosus remains open for over 3 months after birth, it is called patent ductus arteriosus. It is the most common extracardiac left-to-right shunt. A young patient with increased pulmonary vascularity and a large aortic knob is a typical radiographic presentation of patent ductus arteriosus. The ductus may calcify. In the rare *aorticopultnonary window*, the shunt is in the ascending aorta and the knob does not enlarge. Pulmonary hypertension is a frequent late complication of an untreated patent ductus arteriosus. |
| **Total anomalous pulmonary venous return (TAPVR) (Fig. 1.48)** | Nonobstructive TAPVR<br>1 If pulmonary veins drain directly into the right atrium the plain film appearance may be identical to the atrial septal defect.<br>2 If there is persistent left vena cava or vena vrticalis, the heart and mediastinum have a number 8 or snowman appearance.<br>3 The hypoplastic aorta and enlarged pulmonary artery form a shelf-like density superimposed on the left abnormal veins.<br>4 The right atrium and right ventricle are dilated. The left heart is hypoplastic. | All venous blood returns to the right atrium, either directly or through a systemic vein (superior or inferior vena cava, portal vein). Atrial septal defect is a life-saving anomaly in this condition. Thus there is a combined left-to-right and right-to-left shunt. Obstruction of the pulmonary vein (e.g., drainage into the portal vein) is associated with pulmonary venous congestion and normal heart size. |
| **Partial anomalous venous return (PAVR) (Fig. 1.33)** | There may be no abnormality in the chest roentgenogram. Hypervascularity, right heart enlargement, and an anomalous vessel crossing downward on the right side of the heart may be present. | PAVR is more common than TAPVR and usually asymptomatic. |

*(continues on page 40)*

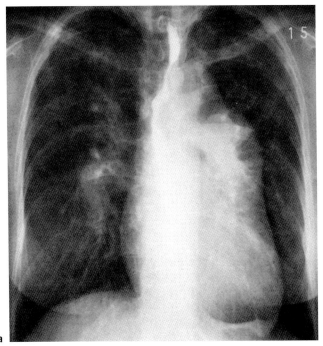
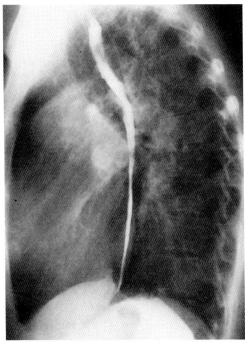

a

b

Fig. 1.**47 a, b**   Patent ductus arteriosus, age 40, with pulmonary arterial hypertension. Very large main pulmonary artery and right hilar shadow. The smaller left hilum is seen through the wide pulmonary artery segment. Left heart is only slightly enlarged.

Fig. 1.**48**   Total anomalous pulmonary venous return with persistent left vena cava, which produces a snowman appearance. Increased pulmonary vasculature.

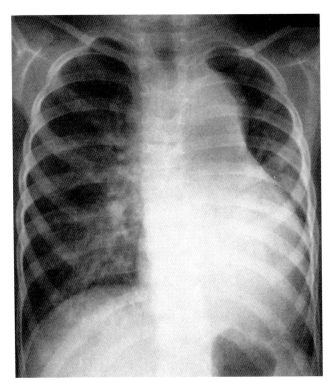

**Table 1.10   (Cont.) Dilatation of the Main Pulmonary Artery Segment**

| Disease | Radiographic Findings | Comments |
|---|---|---|
| **Isolated pulmonary stenosis (see also coarctation of the pulmonary arteries) (Fig. 1.49)** | In the majority of cases the chest findings are entirely normal except for the prominence of the main pulmonary artery.<br>The left pulmonary artery is often more enlarged than the right. | Pulmonary stenosis may occur in *rubeola syndrome* (transplacental infection), *carcinoid syndrome*, or *rheumatic heart disease*.<br>Congenital pulmonary valvular stenosis is a relatively common anomaly. Poststenotic dilatation of the pulmonary arterial segment is absent in the less common *infundibular* pulmonary stenosis (5 % of pulmonary stenoses). |
| **Pulmonary stenosis with atrial septal defect (Fallot's trilogy)** | A prominent main pulmonary segment associated with pulmonary oligemia. This is an important sign to differentiate Fallot's trilogy from tetralogy of Fallot, pseudotruncus arteriosus, and tricuspid atresia.<br>Secondary tricuspid insufficiency following right ventricular enlargement may enlarge the right atrium. The pulmonary valve calcification is rarely seen. | In most cases of pulmonary stenosis there is an open foramen ovale, less frequently a true atrial septal defect. Pulmonary stenosis associated with a ventricular septal defect is usually called tetralogy of Fallot even if the aorta may not be overriding. |
| **Mitral valve disease Tricuspid atresia Truncus arteriosus (type I, common origin of aorta and pulmonary artery)** | Enlargement of the main pulmonary artery segment occurs in these conditions. | These entities are discussed in Tables 1.**6** and 1.**7**. |
| **Congenital coronary fistula** | Plain films reveal a nonspecific left-to-right shunt with prominent pulmonary artery segment, dilated pulmonary vessels and a dilated left atrium. The aortic knob is normal. | A communication between a coronary vessel and a cardiac chamber or a pulmonary artery. The right coronary artery is more commonly involved and usually terminates in the right heart or pulmonary trunk. |
| **Cor triatriatum sinistrum** | Plain roentgenographic findings are not characteristic, but include: Prominent main pulmonary artery segment Prominent hilar vessels Enlargement of the right ventricle Occasionally there is pulmonary venous congestion and rarely left atrial enlargement | A transverse incomplete fibromuscular membrane divides the left atrium into two chambers with a hemodynamic effect similar to that of mitral stenosis. Patent foramen ovale and atrial septal defect are commonly associated. |
| **Common atrioventricular canal (Endocardial cushion defect)** | Cardiomegaly with findings indicative of a nonspecific left-to-right shunt. Pulmonary hypertension often develops in adults. | Different combinations of ostium primum atrial septal defect, cleft mitral and/or tricuspidal valves and ventricular septal defect occur. Pulmonary stenosis is a common associated anomaly. |
| **Coarctation of pulmonary arteries** | An unusual combination of small hilar arteries and large posthilar central branches is suggestive of this diagnosis. An associated pulmonary valvular stenosis is present in over half of the cases. | A rare anomaly in which single or multiple constrictions occur in the branches of the pulmonary artery. The vessels immediately distal to the narrowing are prominent because of poststenotic dilatation. |

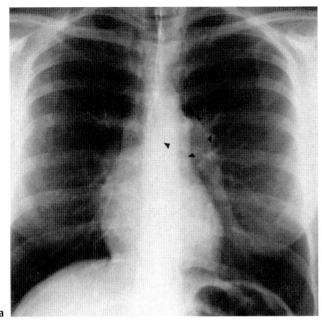

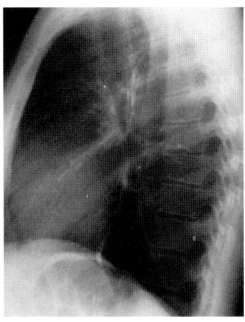

a

b

Fig. 1.**49 a, b**    Isolated pulmonary valvular stenosis, **a** Heart size and pulmonary vascularity are normal, but the main pulmonary artery and its left main branch are enlarged in the PA projection, **b** The lateral film only shows some prominence of the anterior heart border (right ventricular hypertrophy).

# 2 Mediastinal or Hilar Enlargement

The mediastinum is defined as the extrapleural space within the thorax lying between the lungs. The soft-tissue structures that compose the margins of the mediastinum and abut against the lungs usually cast discernible shadows on roentgenograms. These lung-mediastinal interfaces are keys to the radiologic analysis of the mediastinum. Well-penetrated high kVp films are essential to visualize the interfaces lying behind the lateral margins of the mediastinum and heart. Opacification of the esophagus may further help in delineating the suspected lesion.

Although careful analysis of the mediastinum on plain films is not a replacement for computed tomography of known or suspected mass lesions, it is important in detecting early or unsuspected lesions from routine chest roentgenograms. Differentiation of mediastinal disease from cardiac, pericardial, pleural, and pulmonary lesions is better done with CT.

*Useful lines and signs* in anteroposterior projection; Fig. 2.1: The *paraspinal line* may be displaced by pleural fluid, a paravertebral abscess, hemorrhage from a dorsal spine fracture, or extravertebral extension of a neoplasm. The more prominent the aorta, the wider the space between the left paraspinal line and the spine. Visualization of *normal paraesophageal* and *posterior junction* lines are due to the lack of interposed soft-tissue or esophageal distention.

The *paratracheal* and *parabronchial lines* become wider (over 2 to 3 mm) with pleural thickening or fluid, mediastin-itis, and hemorrhages. An uneven outline is likely due to paratracheal lymphadenopathy or tumor. The normal azygos vein is seen as a spindle shaped dense widening of the right paratracheobronchial line at the level of the tracheal bifurcation, and its transverse diameter may vary with posture and Valsalva maneuver, which can be used to differentiate the azygos vein from an enlarged lymph node. In upright position it is normally less than one centimeter wide. Increased systemic venous pressure (congestive heart failure, acute pulmonary hypertension due to embolism, constrictive pericarditis), portal thrombosis, ascending thrombosis of the vena cava, or absence of the subhepatic portion of the vena cava, may cause dilatation of the azygos vein.

The anterior borders of the upper lobes join immediately behind the manubrium to form the *anterior junction line* slightly to the left of midline. It is not seen in infants and young children because of the presence of the thymus. Enlargement of the aorta, hemorrhage, adenopathy, or tumor may interpose between the lungs at this point.

On the left side the paraesophageal line is not consistently visualized, but the *para-aortic* line is continuous with the profile of the aortic arch. This line is often curved due to elongation of the aorta. A discontinuity may represent coarctation of the aorta (Fig. 1.40). Coarctation may also cause convexity of the profile of the left subclavian artery above the aortic knob. The angles between the aorta and the subclavian artery as well as the indentation between the

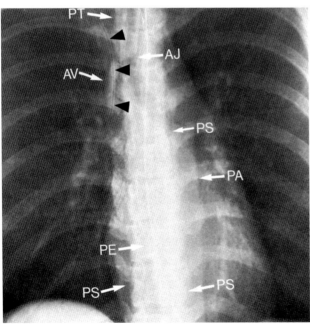

Fig. 2.1a **Mediastinal lines** as seen in anteroposterior projection. The location of superior vena cava, trachea, and esophagus are demonstrated by a CVP line and tracheal and esophageal tubes. PT = paratracheal line, AV azygos vein, AJ anterior junction line, PS = paraspinal line, PA para-aortic line, PE paraesophageal line. Central venous catheter (arrow heads).

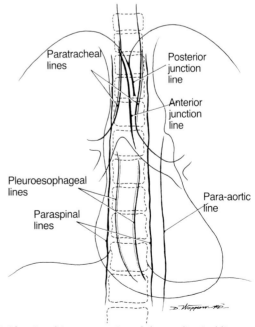

Fig. 2.1b Graphic presentation of the mediastinal lines.

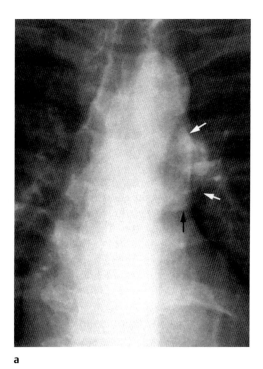

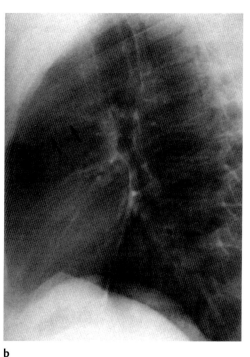

Fig. 2.**2 a, b Hilum overlay sign, a** A double profile of the main pulmonary artery segment, which appears enlarged (arrows), **b** Lateral film shows that there is a mass (lymphoma) in the anterior mediastinum (arrow), which projects over the left hilum in posteroanterior projection.

a        b

aorta and the superior surface of the pulmonary artery may be obliterated by lymphadenopathy or tumor. A double profile of the main pulmonary artery segment, if not explained by the left main artery, is likely due to a neoplasm, usually anterior to the pulmonary artery (*hilum overlay sign*, Fig. 2.**2**).

Widening of the whole mediastinum in anteroposterior projection and disappearance of the normal mediastinopulmonary interfaces occurs especially in hemorrhage and in *postoperative bleeding*, but it may occur with extensive infiltrating *neoplasm*, mediastinal *amyloidosis*, mediastinal *fibrosis*, and *inflammation*. Since the cephalic border of the anterior portion of the mediastinum ends at the level of the clavicles while that of the posterior portion extends much higher, a lesion clearly visible above the clavicles on the frontal view must lie entirely within the thorax. The more cephalad an upper mediastinal mass extends while still remaining visible, the more posteriorly it lies. A thoracic lesion in anatomic contact with the neck or extending into it will be obliterated along its upper lateral borders by the cervical soft tissues (*cervicothoracic sign*, Fig. 2.**3**). Thoracoabdominal mass lesions may be visible through the diaphragm, since they are in contact with the posterior lower lobes. Lack of downward convergence of the lower border of such a lesion (*iceberg sign*, Fig. 2.**4**) indicates that a considerable portion of the mass is in the abdomen. An iceberg sign is common in thoracoabdominal *aneurysms, esophagogastric lesions*, and *azygos continuations of the inferior vena cava*. Also, a *retroperitoneal tumor* may extend into the thorax and widen the inferior paravertebral shadow.

In about 9% of infants and young children the normal thymus may produce a *sail shadow* projecting from the upper mediastinum on the frontal film (Fig. 2.**5**). The sail shadow is differentiated from right upper lobe consolidation by its well defined vertical lateral border, and from encapsulated pleural effusion by its sharp inferior angle. The lateral borders of the normal thymus may be indented by adjacent ribs, causing a subtle wavy margin on the frontal projection that is not seen in thymic tumors or in other anterior mediastinal masses. In an infant, *pneumomediastinum* may dis-

sect the thymus from the rest of the mediastinum and elevate it like a 'spinnaker sail.'

If a thymus in the neonate less than 4 days of age is not visible in anteroposterior or lateral radiographs of the chest (the retrosternal area is lucent, the anterior borders of the heart and great vessels are clearly defined, and in the frontal projection the mediastinum is narrow), thymic aplasia should be suspected. Absence of the thymus and parathyroids (immunologic deficiency and tetany) is called *DiGeorge syndrome* (Fig. 2.**6**). Hypoplastic mandible, deformities of the ear and anomalies of the aortic arch may be associated. Thymic aplasia or hypoplasia may be seen also in severe, *combined immunodeficiency syndromes.*

In lateral view, the mediastinum also has significant profiles (Fig. 2.**7**). Effacement of the aortic arch and tracheal wall profiles indicates interposed soft tissue. The *posterior tracheal band* is a 3-mm-wide band extending from the upper mediastinum to the lower lobe bronchi. It is well visualized in patients who have a sizable azygoesophageal recess filled by the right lung. *Carcinoma of the esophagus*, other *mediastinal neoplasms, bleeding*, or *infection* may obliterate a previously well-visualized posterior tracheal band or cause its general or localized widening (Fig. 2.**8**). The posterior margin of the inferior vena cava is always seen in good-quality lateral films. Its absence is rare (Fig. 2.**9**).

Differentiation of enlarged hilar blood vessels from hilar lymph adenopathy may be easier if one remembers that blood vessels tend to be parallel with bronchi, whereas lymph nodes actually surround them and may produce accentuated cross-sectional shadows of main bronchi in the lateral view. Mediastinal contrast enhanced CT greatly helps differentiation of blood vessels from other structures.

The lines and signs presented above are helpful in localizing a lesion. Division of the mediastinum into anterior, middle, and posterior mediastina is more useful than strictly anatomical subdivision. This artificial division of the mediastinum into anterior, middle, and posterior portions varies among different authors. The division used in this presentation is shown in Fig. 2.**10**. The shape, size, and radiographic structure of mediastinal mass lesions in conventional films

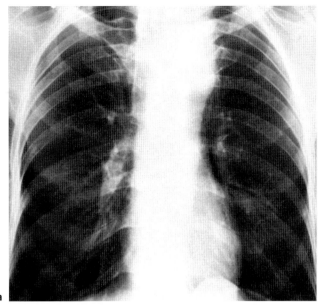

a

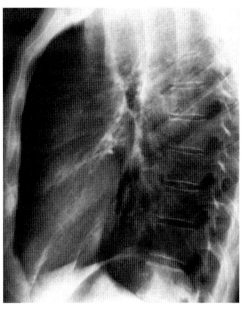

b

Fig. 2.**3 a, b   Cervicothoracic sign, a** In frontal projection, the upper mediastinal mass extends over the clavicles and joins into the soft tissues of the neck, indicating posterior position of the

mass, as shown also in **b** by the lateral film. Carcinoma of the esophagus.

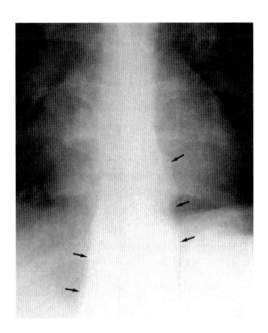

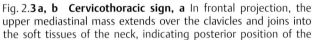

Fig. 2.**4   Iceberg sign.** Nodular widening of the paraver tebral soft tissues (arrows), more so on the left. Para-aortic metastases of a testicular carcinoma extending beyond the diaphragm.

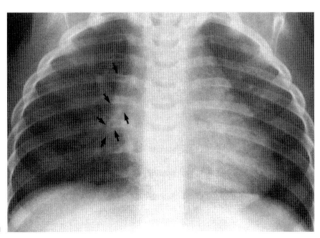

a

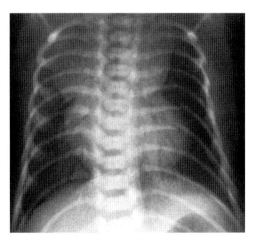

b

Fig. 2.**5 a, b**   Thymic sail shadow, **a** A small "sail" that has a well-defined border and sharp inferior angle (arrows), **b** Thymus pre-

senting as an upper mediastinal mass with a sharp inferior angle on the right side.

often provide insufficient information for definitive diagnosis and computed tomography is required for better anatomical definition. Different types of lesions tend to occur at different anteroposterior subdivisions of the mediastinum. Associated pulmonary or pleural changes provide further information for differential diagnosis.

The most common lesions which cause mediastinal widening are summarized in Table 2.1 according to their usual location. Enlarged lymph nodes in this context refer to masses which are recognizable on plain radiographs, on which normal-sized lymph nodes are not seen unless they are calcified. The question of how to define the boundary between normal and enlarged individual lymph nodes, commonly encountered in CT or more resently in PET-CT, will therefore not be discussed. In Table 2.2, diseases which cause hilar and/or mediastinal lymph node enlargement are discussed, while diseases causing diffuse mediastinal widening are presented in Table 2.3.

**Table 2.1  The Most Common Lesions in the Anterior, Middle and Posterior Mediastinum**

| Anterior Mediastinum | Middle Mediastinum | Posterior Mediastinum |
|---|---|---|
| Aneurysm of ascending aorta | Aneurysm of aortic arch | *Aneurysm or tortuosity of descending aorta* |
| *Lymphoma* (most common) | Azygos vein enlargement | (most common) |
| Pericardial cyst | Bronchogenic cyst | Lymph node enlargement |
| Retrosternal thyroid | Esophageal lesions | Neurogenic tumor |
| Teratoid lesion | Hiatal hernia | Paraspinal manifestations of spinal lesions |
| Thymic lesion | *Lymph node enlargement* (most common) | |
| | Thyroid tumor | |
| | (Hilar vascular dilatation) | |

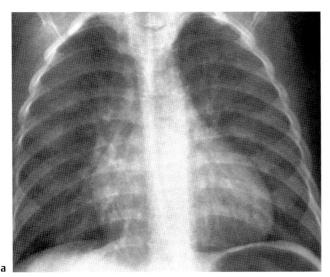

a

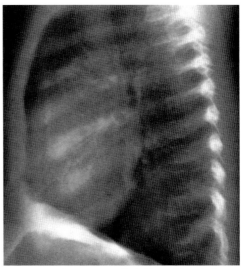

b

Fig. 2.**6 a, b   DiGeorge syndrome.** Absence of thymus is suggested **a** by the narrow upper mediastinum, presence of the ante-

rior junction line in a small child, and **b** radiolucency of the retrosternal space in the lateral view.

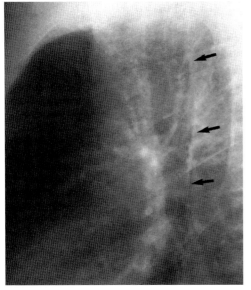

Fig. 2.**7   Normal posterior tracheal band** (arrows)

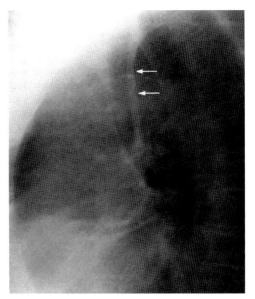

Fig. 2.**8   Thickening of the posterior tracheal band** (arrows).

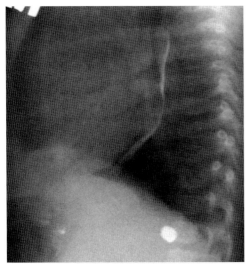

Fig. 2.**9   Congenital absence of the proximal IVC.** The silhouette of the inferior vena cava, normally present in the lateral film, is lacking. Blood is conducted via the azygos vein.

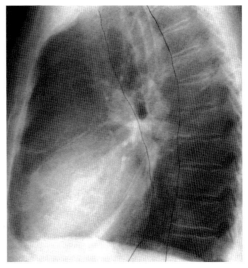

Fig. 2.**10   Division of the mediastinum** into three (artificial) compartments. "Anterior mediastinum" refers to front of the trachea or of the posterior cardiac silhouette. "Posterior mediastinum" refers to area posterior to the anterior paraspinal line. "Middle mediastinum" refers to the compartment between these two artificial lines.

### Table 2.2    Hilar and/or Mediastinal Lymph Node Enlargement

| Disease | Radiographic Findings | Comments |
|---|---|---|
| **Neoplastic diseases (malignant or benign)** | | |
| **Bronchogenic carcinoma (Fig. 2.11)** | Unilateral hilar node enlargement involving bronchopulmonary and tracheobronchial nodes, in some cases paratracheal and posterior mediastinal nodes. | Influence of cell type:<br>1  A hilar mass as the sole roentgenographic abnormality is characteristic of an undifferentiated small-cell carcinoma;<br>2  Generalized mediastinal widening almost certainly indicates spread from an undifferentiated carcinoma;<br>3  Hilar or mediastinal lymph node enlargement is rare in *alveolar cell* (bronchiolar) *carcinoma*. |
| **Hodgkin's disease (Fig. 2.12)** | Bilateral but asymmetric enlargement, especially of paratracheal and tracheobronchial nodes, frequently also anterior mediastinal and retrosternal nodes. Bronchopulmonary nodes are less frequently enlarged than the more central ones. Unilateral involvement is very rare. | Mediastinal lymph node enlargement is seen on the initial chest roentgenogram in approximately 50% of patients. May be associated with pulmonary involvement or pleural effusion in advanced cases. |
| **Non-Hodgkin's lymphoma** | Bilateral, asymmetric node enlargement similar to Hodgkin's disease. | May occasionally present as parenchymal consolidation without associated lymph node enlargement. |
| **Leukemia** | Usually symmetric enlargement of mediastinal and bronchopulmonary nodes. | Occurs in 25% of patients, more commonly in lymphocytic than in myelocytic leukemia. Pleural effusion and parenchymal involvement may be associated. |

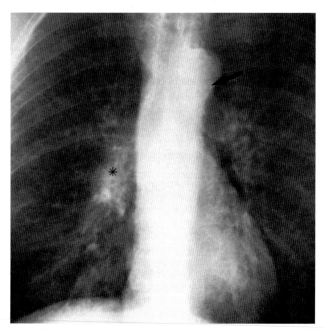

Fig. 2.**11**  **Small cell carcinoma** with mediastinal lymph node metastases and lymphangitis carcinomatosa. Enlarged right tracheobronchial lymph nodes (asterisk) and subtle obliteration of the notch between aorta and main pulmonary artery by metastatic lymph nodes (arrow).

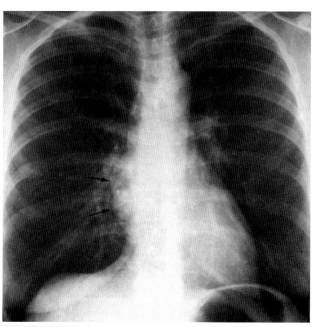

Fig. 2.**12**  **Hodgkin's disease.** Enlarged anterior mediastinal and hilar lymph nodes. Intrapulmonary mass lesion in the left lung.

Fig. 2.**13 a–d**  **Bronchopulmonary amyloidosis. a, b** Hilar and ▷ azygos nodes are enlarged, with a pattern similar to sarcoidosis. Even small pulmonary densities occur, **c, d** The same patient, 6 years later. Unlike sarcoidosis, the hilar and mediastinal lymph nodes continually grow. Miliary parenchymal changes have also increased.

### Table 2.2  (Cont.) Hilar and/or Mediastinal Lymph Node Enlargement

| Disease | Radiographic Findings | Comments |
|---|---|---|
| Immunoblastic lymph-adenopathy (a hyperimmune disorder of B lymphocytes) | Bilateral, asymmetric node enlargement similar to Hodgkin's disease. | Lungs are occasionally affected in a pattern similar to Hodgkin's disease. |
| Heavy-chain disease (a plasma cell dyscrasia) | Symmetric enlargement of mediastinal lymph nodes. | Hepatosplenomegaly is common, lung involvement rare. |
| Bronchopulmonary amyloidosis (a plasma cell dyscrasia) (Fig. 2.13) | Symmetric hilar and mediastinal lymph node enlargement. Enlarged nodes may be densely calcified. | Sometimes associated with diffuse pulmonary involvement. |

(continues on page 50)

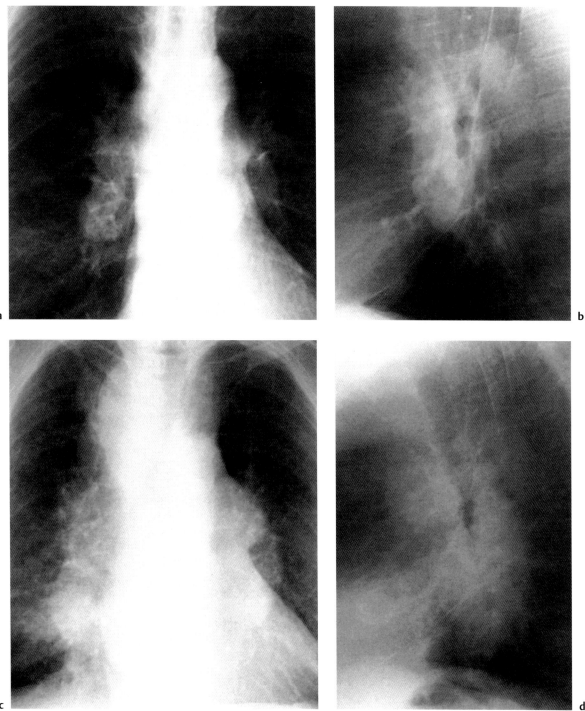

a

b

c

d

**Table 2.2   (Cont.) Hilar and/or Mediastinal Lymph Node Enlargement**

| Disease | Radiographic Findings | Comments |
|---|---|---|
| Lymph node metastases (Fig. 2.14) | Unilateral or bilateral enlargement of either hilar or mediastinal nodes or both. | May be associated with lymphangitic changes in the lungs (see Table 2.3). |
| Castleman's disease (giant lymph node hyperplasia) | hilar or mediastinal nodes or both. Large circumscribed mediastinal mass is the most common presentation. | lymphangitic changes in the lungs (see Table 2.3). This rare benign condition may be associated with fever, anemia and gammaglobulinemia. Two types can be differentiated. Type 1: the hyaline vascular type (90%), almost always local, with no systemic symptoms; Type 2 the plasma-cell type, which may be multicentric and associated with systemic symptoms. |
| **Bacterial and myco-plasma infections** | | |
| Primary tuberculosis (Fig. 2.15) | Mostly unilateral hilar (60%) or hilar and paratracheal (40%) lymph node enlargement. Bilateral node enlargement is a rare presentation. | Hilar node enlargement differentiates primary tuberculosis from secondary (reunification) tuberculosis. In the latter, there is no observable lymphadenopathy. |
| Tularemia (Francisella tularensis) | Unilateral hilar node enlargement with characteristically oval pneumonic consolidations and pleural effusion. | Ipsilateral hilar node enlargement occurs in 25–50% of tularemic pneumonias. Is a potential bioterrorism agent. |
| Pertussis (whooping cough) | Unilateral hilar node enlargement. | Often associated with ipsilateral segmental pneumonia and atelectasis. |
| Anthrax (Bacillus anthracis) | Symmetric enlargement of all lymph nodes or generalized mediastinal widening. | Often associated with pleural effusion, rarely with pulmonary hemorrhages. Has been used as a bioterrorism weapon |
| Plague pneumonia (caused by Yersinia pestis) | Symmetric hilar and paratracheal node enlargement. | Nonsegmental homogeneous consolidations may occur in lungs mimicking alveolar edema. May be used as a bioterrorism weapon. |
| Mycoplasma pneumoniae | Unilateral or bilateral hilar lymphnode enlargement associated with segmental pneumonia, predominantly in lower lobes. | Most common in children. Together with parenchymal disease. |
| Viral, rickettsial infections | Unilateral or bilateral hilar node enlargement. | |
| Rubeola | Bilateral hilar node enlargement may be associated with diffuse interstitial pneumonia. | If pneumonia in rubeola is segmental, it is due to secondary bacterial infection. |
| Echovirus pneumonia | Bilateral hilar node enlargement and associated increase of bronchovascular markings. | Respiratory infections occur predominantly in infants. |
| Varicella pneumonia | Bilateral hilar node enlargement associated with patchy, diffuse air-space consolidation. | Pulmonary consolidation may mask hilar node reaction. Mainly occurs in adults with varicella. |
| Psittacosis (ornithosis) | Unilateral or bilateral hilar node enlargement associated with variable radiographic presentations of pneumonia. | Roentgenographic resolution of pneumonia is slow. |
| Epstein-Barr (infectious mononucleosis) (Fig. 2.16) | Bilateral, symmetric, predominantly hilar lymph node enlargement. | Splenomegaly. Roentgenographic changes in the lungs are rare. |
| AIDS (acquired immunodeficiency syndrome) (Figs. 2.15, 2.17) | Bilateral lymph node enlargement. | Lymphadenopathy is a common finding in AIDS patients (up to 80%). Lymphadenopathy is most often related to chest infections, less commonly caused by AIDS-associated lymphoma. |

*(continues on page 52)*

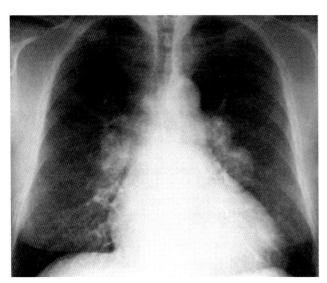

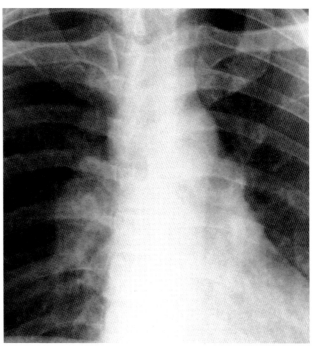

Fig. 2.**14**  **Metastatic melanoma** with lymphangitis carcinomatosa and bilateral hilar lymph node enlargement.

Fig. 2.**15**  **Primary tuberculosis** in a patient with AIDS. Right hilar lymph node enlargement.

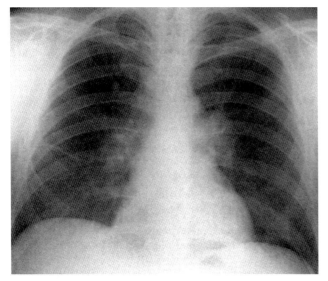

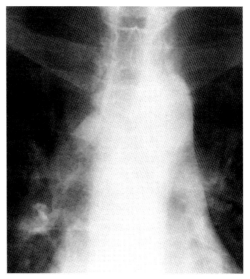

Fig. 2.**16**  **Infectious mononucleosis.** Enlargement of bronchopulmonary nodes and the azygos node – a pattern characteristic of sarcoidosis.

Fig. 2.**17**  Benign mediastinal lymphadenopathy in **AIDS.** Lymph nodes on the right side are predominantly enlarged, both in the hilar and the upper mediastinal regions.

**Table 2.2 (Cont.) Hilar and/or Mediastinal Lymph Node Enlargement**

| Disease | Radiographic Findings | Comments |
|---|---|---|
| **Fungal infections** | | |
| **Histoplasmosis (Fig. 2.18)** | Unilateral or bilateral, hilar, mediastinal, and occasionally intrapulmonary lymph node enlargement, with or sometimes without associated pneumonia. Hilar node enlargement is a common feature in all other fungal infections, too. | *Several forms of presentation:*<br>1 Benign type: one or more ill-defined non-segmental opacities in lungs,<br>2 Pneumonic type: simulates an acute non-segmental air-space pneumonia of bacterial origin,<br>3 Histoplasmoma: one or few "coin" lesions, which may calcify ("target" lesion). Hilar lymph node calcification is common, although nodes may not be enlarged,<br>4 Lymph node enlargement without associated pulmonary changes, particulary common in children,<br>5 Acute diffuse nodular histoplasmosis with or without pulmonary manifestations (pneumonia or miliary nodules). |
| **Coccidioidomycosis** | Unilateral or bilateral enlargement of hilar and/or paratracheal nodes, with or without associated pulmonary parenchymal disease. | Enlargement of paratracheal lymph nodes may indicate an imminent dissemination. |
| **Sporotrichosis** | Unilateral hilar node enlargement. | The associated parenchymal changes are variable. |
| **Parasitic diseases** | | |
| **Tropical eosinophilia (caused by filariasis)** | Occasionally bilateral hilar lymph node enlargement. | Micronodular densities and increased linear markings in the lungs. |
| **Pneumoconiosis** | | |
| **Silicosis (Fig. 2.19)** | Symmetric, predominantly bronchopulmonary lymph node enlargement, usually associated with diffuse nodular disease of the parenchyma. Eggshell calcification of lymph nodes occurs in 5% of silicosis patients. | When present, eggshell calcification of lymph nodes is almost pathognomonic of silicosis. Occasionally it is seen in sarcoidosis and irradiated Hodgkin's disease. Lymph node enlargement is present in some cases of *coal miner's lung*. |
| **Chronic berylliosis** | Symmetric bronchopulmonary lymph node enlargement occurs in a minority of cases, | The roentgenographic pattern in chest varies and is neither specific nor diagnostic. |
| **Other diseases** | | |
| **Sarcoidosis (Fig. 2.20) (The most common cause of bilateral hilar node enlargement)** | Symmetric enlargement of bronchopulmonary, tracheobronchial and paratracheal lymph nodes is characteristically seen in 75% to 90% of patients. The outer borders of the enlarged hila are usually lobulated and there is often a lucent zone between the heart and enlarged tracheobronchial nodes. Enlargement of the azygos node is also typical. | Typical patterns are:<br>1 Lymph node enlargement without pulmonary abnormality<br>2 Combined diffuse pulmonary disease and lymph node enlargement (in up to 20%)<br>3 Homogeneous alveolar-looking densities (rare)<br>4 Uneven pulmonary fibrosis.<br>With the onset of diffuse lung disease, the lymph node size diminishes, which aids in differentiating sarcoidosis from lymphoma and tuberculosis. |
| **Extrinsic allergic alveolitis (occupational exposure to organic dust <5 μm in size)** | Rarely a combination of symmetric enlargement of bronchopulmonary nodes associated with diffuse interstitial pattern. | May mimic sarcoidosis, but hilar node enlargement in extrinsic allergic alveolitis is rare except for mushroom-worker's lung, where it is fairly common. |

*(continues on page 54)*

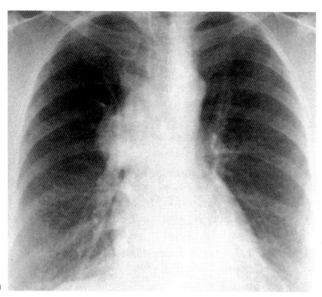 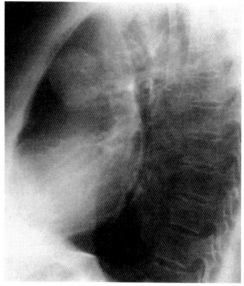

a                                                                                            b

Fig. 2.**18**  **Calcified histoplasmoma** of the right anterior mediastinum. Hilar nodes are not enlarged.

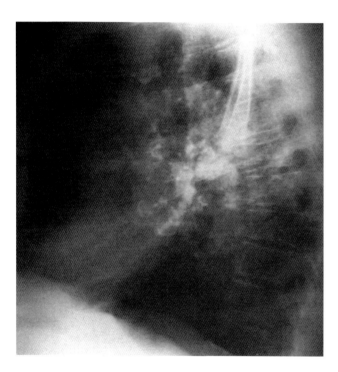

Fig. 2.**19**  **Sillcosis.** Enlarged hilar and mediastinal lymph nodes with eggshell calcification.

Fig. 2.**20a, b**  **Sarcoidosis.** Characteristic distribution of lymph node enlargement: bronchopulmonary and tracheobronchial nodes (including the azygos node) leaving a lucent zone between the nodes and the heart.
▽

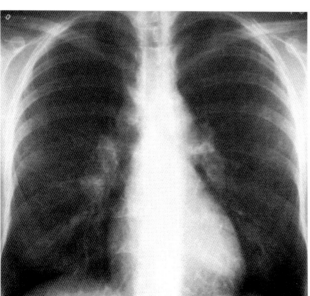 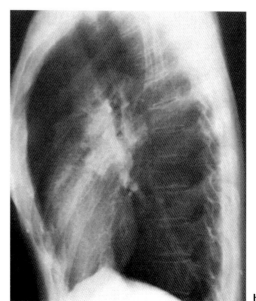

a                                                                                            b

### Table 2.2    (Cont.) Hilar and/or Mediastinal Lymph Node Enlargement

| Disease | Radiographic Findings | Comments |
|---|---|---|
| Langerhans'-cell histiocytosis (Histiocytosis X) | Symmetric hilar and mediastinal lymph node enlargement is a rare manifestation of Langerhans'-cell histiocytosis. | Lymph node enlargement in the presence of diffuse interstitial pulmonary disease favors sarcoidosis. |
| Goodpasture syndrome | Symmetric hilar node enlargement occurs predominantly in the acute stage. | The degree of diffuse alveolar and interstitial disease is dependent on the number of hemorrhagic episodes. |
| Cystic fibrosis (Fig. 2.21) | Unilateral or bilateral hilar node enlargement occurs in about half of chest X-rays of adult patients with cystic fibrosis. Can resemble sarcoidosis or lymphoma. | Areas of atelectasis and bronchiectasis with diffuse increase of pulmonary markings, hyperinflation, and pulmonary arterial hypertension predominate. |
| Drug induced | Bilateral hilar or mediastinal lymph node enlargement. | May occur during diphenylhydantoin or trimethadione therapy. |
| Pseudoenlargement | Enlargement of hilar vascular shadows may mimic hilar adenopathy. Blood vessels tend to parallel the bronchi, lymph nodes surround them. | Seen often in cardiovascular diseases (e.g., shunts, cardiac failure, valvular pulmonic stenosis, cor pulmonale, pulmonary embolism). |

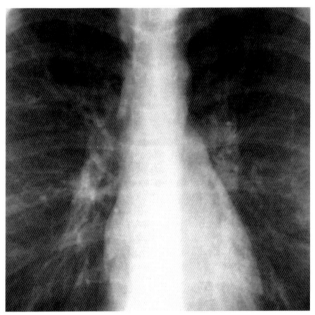 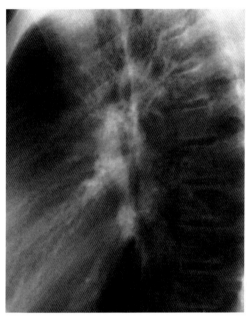

a          b

Fig. 2.**21 a, b   Cystic fibrosis,** age 14. Hilar lymph nodes appear enlarged, but most of the increased density may be vascular, as shown by the lateral view. Pulmonary parenchymal changes are evident.

## Table 2.3   Mediastinal Widening

| Disease | Radiographic Findings | Comments |
|---|---|---|
| **Mediastinal pseudo-widening** | Expiratory film. Scoliosis. | Apparent mediastinal widening in expiratory films occurs especially in infants and children. |
| **Normal thymus** (Fig. 2.5) | Anterior mediastinal mass in a neonate. | For differential diagnostic characteristics, see the introductory text of this chapter. |
| **Foregut cysts (bronchogenic, neurenteric, etc.)** (Fig. 2.22) | Round or oval, usually single well-defined density but can be multilocular. *Bronchogenic* cysts are usually found in contact with the trachea or central bronchi. Rarely they contain air. *Neurenteric* cysts are located in the posterior mediastinum. | Bronchogenic cyst may slowly grow and compress tracheobronchial tree or esophagus. Cysts in the hilar area are usually asymptomatic. Neurenteric cysts are frequently associated with spinal anomalies. The cystic structure of the mass is demonstrated with contrast enhanced CT. |
| **Mesothelial cyst (pericardial or pleuropericardial cysts and diverticula)** (Fig. 1.30) | Smoothly marginated, round or oval density in the anterior or middle mediastinum , most commonly in the right pericardiophrenic angle. | Lateral bulge and smooth, sharp contour differentiate a cyst from right middle lobe lesion or fat in the cardiophrenic angle. Better definition is achieved with CT. |

*(continues on page 56)*

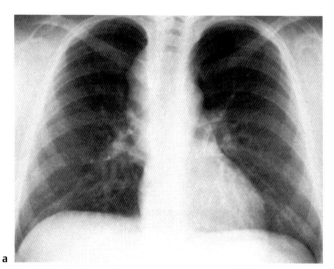
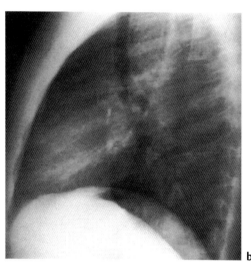

a    b

Fig. 2.**22 a, b**   **Bronchogenic cyst.** An oval well-delineated mass in the right middle mediastinum with anterior tracheal displacement.

### Table 2.3   (Cont.) Mediastinal Widening

| Disease | Radiographic Findings | Comments |
|---|---|---|
| **Diverticula of the pharynx or esophagus (Fig. 2.23)** | A cyst-like structure near pharynx or esophagus. Communication with esophagus is demonstrated by barium swallow. | Small diverticula are not visible without barium. Larger cysts may displace contiguous esophagus. Aspiration pneumonia may be a complication of a pharyngeal diverticulum (Zenker's diverticulum). |
| **Meningocele** | A sharply circumscribed, solitary or multiple density in the posterior mediastinum. | Spine or rib deformities are frequent. |
| Tumors | | |
| **Thyroid masses and tumors (Figs. 2.24, 2.25)** | A smooth or lobulated mass usually in the superior, anterior mediastinum, but may protrude behind the trachea and esophagus. Sometimes calcified. | Calcifications occur both in benign and malignant thyroid masses. Respiratory symptoms and dysphagia may occur. |
| **Thymoma (Figs. 2.26, 2.27)** | Smooth or lobulated anterior mediastinal lesion, rarely calcifies. | Myasthenia gravis is frequently associated. Thyroid and thymic tumors are often roentgenographically indistinguishable. The site of origin is better predicted using CT. |

*(continues on page 58)*

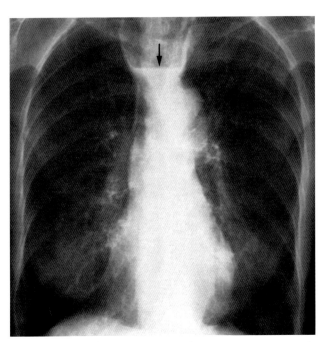

Fig. 2.**23**   **A large Zenker's diverticulum** presenting as a cystic expansion of the upper mediastinum with an air-fluid level (arrow).

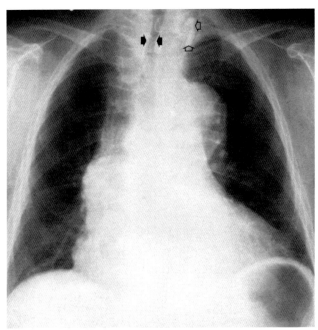

Fig. 2.**24**   **Enlarged thyroid.** Upper mediastinal mass with narrowed trachea (closed arrowheads) and calcification (open arrowheads). The ascending aorta is seen as a hump overlying the right hilus.

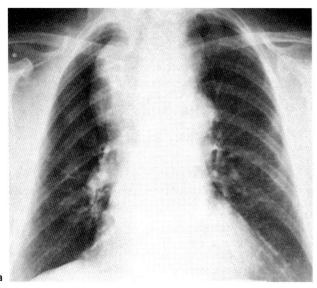
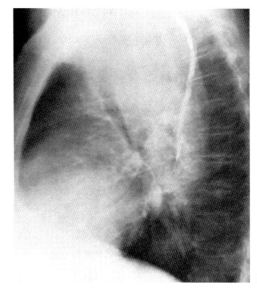

Fig. 2.**25 a, b    Large thyroid** presenting as an upper mediastinal mass,

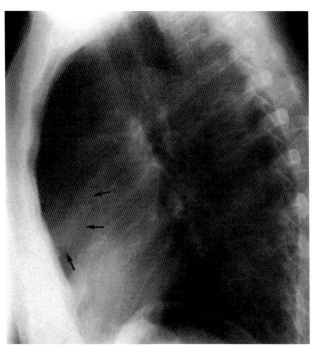

Fig. 2.**26    Thymoma.** A smooth anterior rnediastinal mass main pulmonary segment in posteroanterior projection, but the lesion is behind the sternum in the lateral view (b).which in the lateral view extends down that was visible only in the lateral view (arrows).

Fig. 2.**27 a, b    a A large thymoma** mimics an enlarged into the middle mediastinum between the trachea and esophagus.
▽

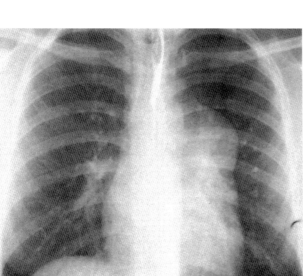
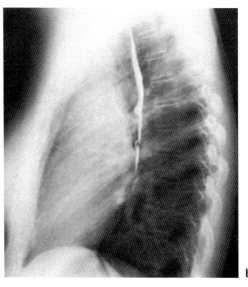

**Table 2.3 (Cont.) Mediastinal Widening**

| Disease | Radiographic Findings | Comments |
|---|---|---|
| **Teratoma Germinal cell neoplasms (dermoid cyst, seminoma, choriocarcinoma, endodermal sinus tumor) (Figs. 2.28, 2.29)** | Smoothly delineated mass, almost invariably in the anterior mediastinum. Calcification, bone, teeth or fat may be identified in teratomas and dermatoid cysts. | Usually manifest in adolescence or early adulthood. Teratomas are most common, they tend to be symptomatic in children. Cystic tumors are usually benign and solid ones malignant. Fat, soft-tissue and bone components are often demonstrated by CT. |
| **Parathyroid tumors** | Most tumors are too small to be seen on plain films, but may be detectable with ultrasound examination. Large ones occur in the anterior, upper mediastinum and may displace the esophagus. | Roentgenographic and laboratory evidence of hyperparathyroidism may be present independent of the size of the tumors. |
| **Lipoma Liposarcoma mediastinal lipomatosis (Fig. 1.31)** | A smooth bulge to either side of the mediastinum, usually anterior. Fat density may be distinguishable even on plain films. CT scans show uniform fat density. | Lipomas are usually asymptomatic. Symmetric widening of the upper mediastinum and large epicardial fat pads (lipomatosis) occurs in long term corticosteroid therapy. |
| **Fibroma Fibrosarcoma Hemangioma hemangiosarcoma hemangioendothelioma, lymphangioma (Fig. 2.30) hygroma leiomyoma (Fig. 2.31)** | Most occur in the anterior mediastinum as well circumscribed densities with no distinctive features. Fibrosarcomas occur more commonly in the posterior mediastinum. | Demonstration of phleboliths is diagnostic of a hemangioma type tumor. Hygroma occurs in infants as a cervicomediastinal mass. |

(continues on page 60)

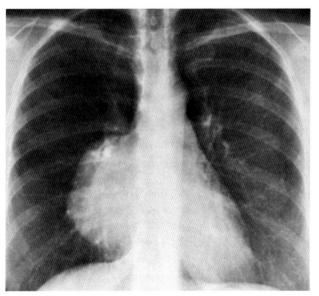
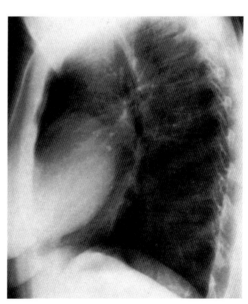

a      b

Fig. 2.**28**   **A large mediastinal teratoma,** radiographically similar to pericardial cyst.

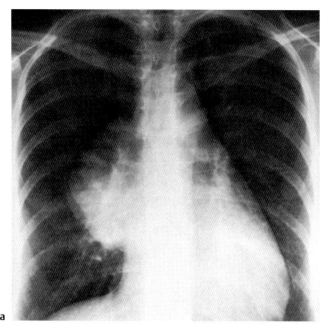
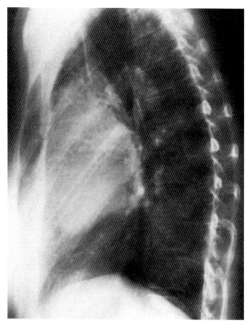

a    b

Fig. 2.**29    Malignant epidermoid tumor** at the right heart border. The tumor is slightly lobulated but otherwise indistinguishable from the teratoma in Fig. 28.

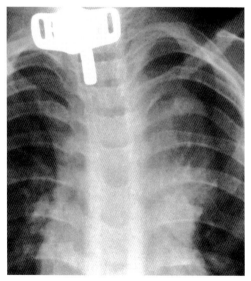

Fig. 2.**30    Cavernous lymphangioma** (cystic hygroma), in a 4-year-old child, appears as a smooth left-sided upper mediastinal mass.

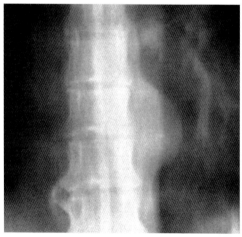

Fig. 2.**31    Paramediastinal leiomyoma.** A smooth bulge attached to the paraspinal ligament without bone erosion.

**Table 2.3 (Cont.) Mediastinal Widening**

| Disease | Radiographic Findings | Comments |
|---|---|---|
| **Lymphoma (Hodgkin's or non-Hodgkin's) Leukemia (Figs. 2.32, 2.33)** | Middle or anterior mediastinal mass. Solitary, tabulated, or symmetrical widening of the mediastinum. Leukemic masses tend to be smaller than those due to lymphoma. | The most common mediastinal mass lesion (25%). Constitutional and local symptoms are frequent, the latter especially in lymphoma. |
| **Metastatic lymph node enlargement (Fig. 2.34)** | Usually in the middle mediastinum, commonly unilateral, involving paratracheal and bronchopulmonary nodes. | The common primary cause is bronchogenic carcinoma. May originate from GI/GU tract (prostate, kidney, etc.). |
| **Esophageal neoplasms (Figs. 2.3 and 2.8)** | Widening of the posterior tracheal band or obliteration of the retrotracheal lucency. Benign tumors are rare (e.g. leiomyoma) and may present as a rounded mass along the course of the esophagus. | Malignant esophageal neoplasms rarely become large enough to be seen as mass lesions, but if the upper two-thirds of 'the esophagus are involved, abnormality of the posterior tracheal band is a fairly sensitive indicator. |

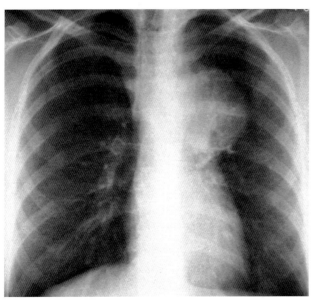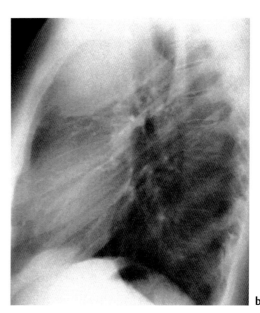

Fig. 2.**32 a, b   Hodgkin's lymphoma.** A solitary anterior mediastinal mass is seen.

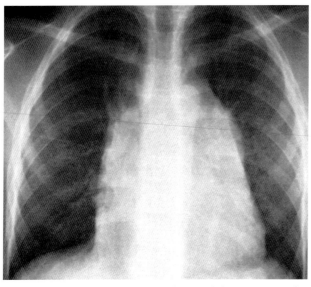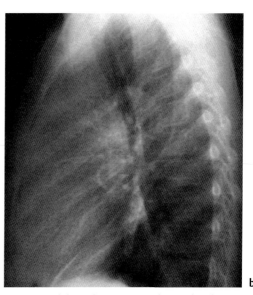

Fig. 2.**33 a, b   Non-Hodgkin's lymphoma** of the anterior mediastinum causing bilateral anterior mediastinal widening.

## Table 2.3   (Cont.) Mediastinal Widening

| Disease | Radiographic Findings | Comments |
|---|---|---|
| **Neurogenic neoplasms:**<br>  neurofibroma (Fig. 2.37,<br>  p. 62)<br>  neurofibrosarcoma<br>  neurilemmoma (Fig. 2.36)<br>  ganglioneuroma (Fig. 2.35)<br>  neuroblastoma<br>  sympathicoblastoma<br>  pheochromocytoma<br>  paraganglioma<br>  chemodectoma | Usually unilateral, round, oval or dumbbell shaped density in the posterior mediastinum. Rib or vertebral erosion associated with a paravertebral lesion is characteristic, but frank destruction occurs only in malignant ones. Pleural effusion or calcification of the tumor may occur.<br>Chemodectomas occur anywhere in the mediastinum. | Almost all neuroblastomas and a few ganglioneuromas produce an excess of catecholamines. Their degradation products (vanillylmandelic acid or metanephrine) are found in the urine. Their demonstration is a sensitive test to diagnose the primary tumor, metastases or recurrencies. |
| **Bone and cartilage neoplasms** | Rounded paravertebral mass associated with possible destruction of affected bone. A rare cause of mediastinal widening. | |

(continues on page 62)

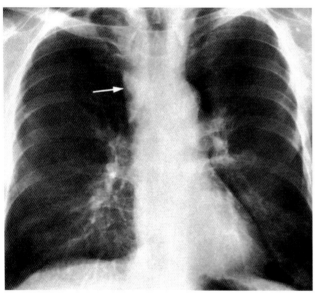

Fig. 2.**34   Metastatic carcinoma** of the larynx. Smooth widening of the upper mediastinum. The azygos node is particularly large (arrow).

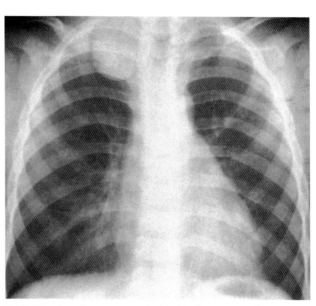

Fig. 2.**35   Ganglioneuroma.** A dumbbell tumor in the superior sulcus, without bone destruction is seen.

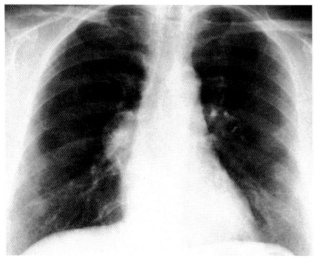
a
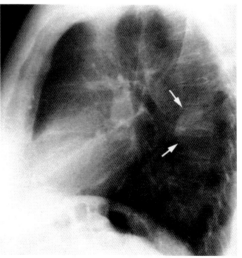
b

Fig. 2.**36 a, b   Neurilemmoma.** A smooth posterior mediastinal mass (arrows), no bone destruction.

**Table 2.3   (Cont.) Mediastinal Widening**

| Disease | Radiographic Findings | Comments |
|---|---|---|
| Castleman's disease (giant lymph node hyperplasia) | A solitary, usually large and sharply circumscribed mass, usually in the middle or posterior mediastinum. | Usually asymptomatic. May occur also in other parts of mediastinum. May represent a "hamartoma" of lymphoid tissue. (See also Table 2.**2**.) |
| Extramedullary hematopoiesis (Fig. 2.38) | Lobulated or smooth, often bilateral paravertebral mass, in a patient with severe anemia and eventual hepatosplenomegaly at the level of the middle and lower thorax. No associated bone lesions are seen. | Extramedullary hematopoiesis occurs most commonly in the congenital hemolytic anemias (*hereditary spherocytosis, thalassemia, sickle cell anemia*). It may occur rarely in other diseases (*myelofibrosis, polycythemia, erythroblastosis fetalis, leukemia, Hodgkin's disease, carcinomatosis, hyperparathyroidism, rickets*) or without a known disease. |
| Chronic granulomatous or sclerosing mediastintis (Figs, 2.39, 2.40) | A lobulated mass, more commonly visible at the right paramediastinal area. Calcification may be present. May occur in any part of mediastinum. | Calcification may not be obvious in plain films, although present in CT. Major airway or superior vena cava compression may be presenting symptoms. May be associated with *tuberculosis* (Fig. 2.**40**) or *sarcoidosis*, or a manifestation of *idiopathic fibrosclerosis* (Fig. 2.**39**). |

*(continues on page 64)*

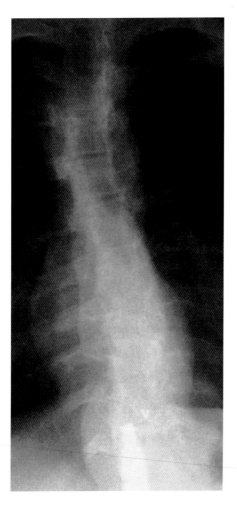

Fig. 2.**37**   **Neurofibromatosls.** Multiple neurofibrornas present as paravertebral masses bilaterally throughout the thoracic spine, which shows rotary scoliosis and erosions.

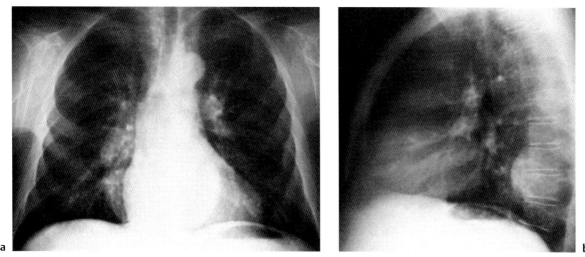

a          b

Fig. 2.**38   Extramedullary hematopoesis** (thalassemia). A smooth paravertebral mass on the left, behind the heart.

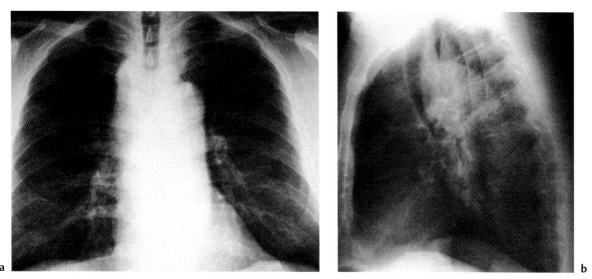

a          b

Fig. 2.**39   Sclerosing mediastinitis.** Bilateral widening of the middle mediastinum, more to the right. The mass compresses the trachea and appears dense because of diffuse calcification.

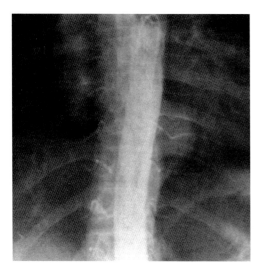

Fig. 2.**40   Tuberculous granuloma.** A smooth paravertebral mass, radiographically indistinguishable from other benign masses in this region (see Fig. 31, page 57). The radiograph was taken during thoracic aortography.

### Table 2.3   (Cont.) Mediastinal Widening

| Disease | Radiographic Findings | Comments |
|---|---|---|
| Acute mediastinitis (Figs. 2.41, 2.42) | Diffuse symmetric widening of mediastinum or a localized mass (abscess), in any part of mediastinum, more commonly in the upper mediastinum. | Most cases are due to esophageal rupture and may show air in mediastinum. CT is sensitive in searching for gas bubbles in the mediastinum. An infection in the neck may spread into the mediastinum. |
| Acute anthrax (*Bacillus anthracis*) | Symmetric widening of mediastinum may be associated with pulmonary hemorrhages, pleural effusion and thickening of bronchovascular bundles. | Most common in sorters and combers in the wool industry. Anthrax has been used as a biological weapon. |
| Vertebral osteomyelitis | Paravertebral mass at the lower mediastinum associated with erosion or destruction of vertebrae. | |
| Aortic aneurysm (Fig. 2.43) | May involve anterior (ascending aorta), middle (aortic arch), or posterior (descending aorta) mediastinum. Saccular dilatation, usually with wall calcification. | See Chapter 1. Contrast enhanced CT is helpful in defining the anatomy of the aneurysm. |
| Dilatation or aneurysm of the innominate artery (right) or the subclavian artery (left) | Smooth lateral bulging above the aorta, in middle mediastinum. | May be associated with atherosclerosis or coarctation of the aorta. May be demonstrated by contrast enhanced CT or with ultrasound through jugular or supraclavicular windows. |
| Aortic arch malformation (Fig. 1.42) | Right aortic arch runs between trachea and esophagus. Usually detected in childhood. | May compress trachea or esophagus. |
| Persistent left superior vena cava (Fig, 2.44) | An accessory vascular "para" line in the frontal view. | Usually present with anomalous pulmonary venous return. |
| Dilatation of pulmonary artery (Fig. 1.43) | Smooth enlargement of the main pulmonary trunk. | See Chapter 1. |

*(continues on page 66)*

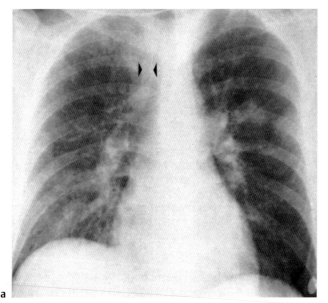
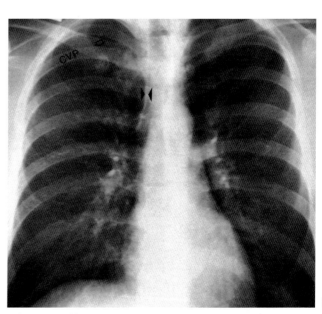

a   b

Fig. 2.**41 a, b**   **Acute mediastinitis,** spreading from a dentogenic abscess, **a** Widening of the mediastinum is best appreciated by observing the width of the paratracheal line (arrowheads). Bilateral pulmonary infiltrates are secondary to shock lung, **b** Normal paratracheal line of the same individual after therapy.

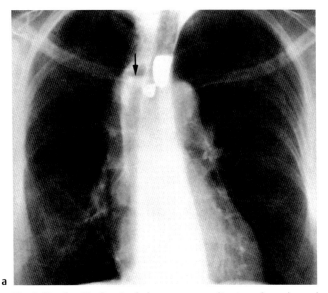

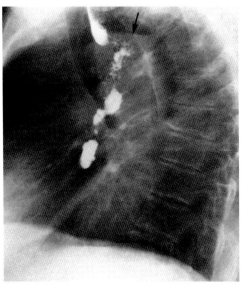

a

b

Fig. 2.**42 a, b    Mediastinal abscess,** a complication of esophageal carcinoma, **a** Widening of mediastinum toward the right. An air-fluid level superimposed on the right clavicle (arrow), **b** Extrae-

sophageal location of the air-fluid level shown with barium in the esophagus.

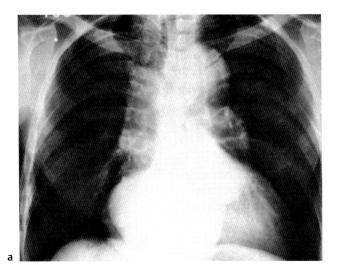

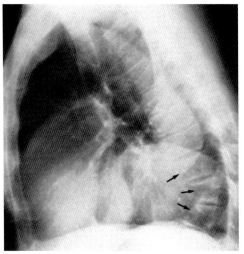

a

b

Fig. 2.**43 a, b    Aneurysm of the thoracic descending aorta** simulating a mediastinal tumor. The aneurysm has eroded three thoracic vertebral bodies anteriorly (T9 to T11, arrows).

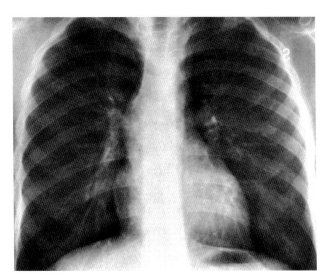

Fig. 2.**44    Persistent left superior vena cava** without other vascular anomalies. An accessory silhouette, continuous with the left heart border and lateral to the aortic shadow (arrows).

**Table 2.3   (Cont.) Mediastinal Widening**

| Disease | Radiographic Findings | Comments |
|---|---|---|
| **Dilatation of the superior vena cava (Fig. 2.45)** | Smooth widening of the right middle paramediastinal area extending from hilum upwards. | Secondary to elevated central venous pressure (heart failure), or compression/obstruction due to a mediastinal mass. |
| **Dilatation of the azygos vein** | A smooth mass at the right tracheobronchial angle. Its diameter changes with change in body position or intrathoracic pressure. | Associated with heart failure, vena cava obstruction, or azygos continuation of the inferior vena cava. |
| **Pneumomediastinum (Fig. 2.46)** | Smooth, usually minor widening of mediastinum associated with air in the mediastinum. Air tends to migrate upward in to the neck. | Commonly spontaneous. May be associated with pneumothorax and subcutaneous or interstitial emphysema. If there is air only in the pericardium, it does not rise above the pulmonary artery: |
| **Mediastinal hemorrhage or hematoma (Fig. 2.47)** | Focal or more commonly diffuse mediastinal widening. | Trauma or mediastinal surgery (most commonly coronary bypass) are the most frequent causes. Rupture of an aortic aneurysm is likely if there is no history of trauma. Hemorrage may be due fracture of thoracic vertebra. |
| **Hernia through foramen of Morgagni** | A round "bump" at the right anterior cardiophrenic angle; can be bilateral. May contain intestine (colon) or liver. | In liver herniation, the abdominal portion of the liver appears small. Congenital cardiac malformation may be associated. |
| **Esophageal hiatus hernia (Fig. 2.48)** | A retrocardiac mass of variable size, usually containing an air-fluid level. | Readily identified by giving a barium swallow. More common in elderly patients. |
| **Herniation through foramen of Bochdalek** | Round or oval retrocardiac density, usually unilateral. 80–90% occur on the left side. If large it may contain bowel loops, which displace ipsilateral lung. | The most common congenital defect of the diaphragm. A large Bochdalek hernia is a rare cause of acute respiratory distress in a neonate. |
| **Diaphragmatic eventration** | A broad-based mass, more laterally on PA chest X-ray than mediastinal lesions. | Usually easy to differentiate from a mediastinal lesion. |
| **Diaphragmatic rupture.** | Usually on the left side after trauma | |

*(continues on page 68)*

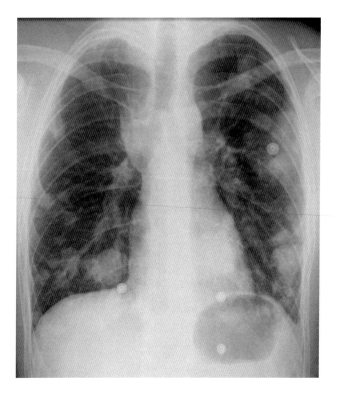

Fig. 2.**45** **Dilatation of superior vena cava** by metastasis of synovial sarcoma of right glenohumeral joint (partially visible) in 28 years old male.

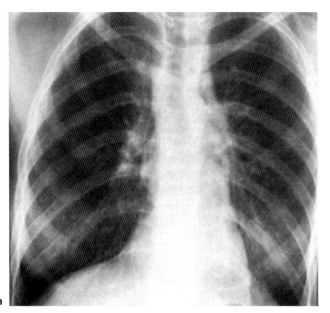
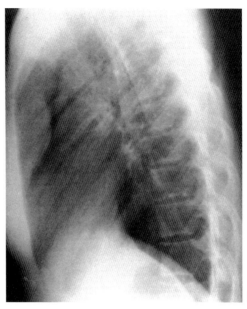

a                                    b

Fig. 2.**46 a, b    Spontaneous pneumomediastinum** in a patient with Hodgkin's disease, **a** Minor widening of the mediastinum in frontal projection, **b** Air outlines the retrosternal mass.

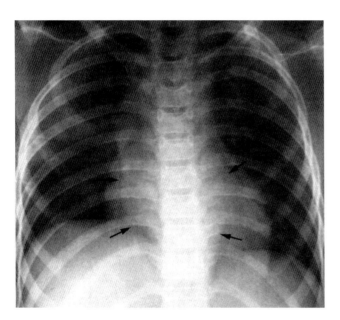

Fig. 2.**47    Traumatic mediastinal hematoma.** Bilateral increase of softtissue density is seen behind the heart (arrows). It does not extend into the posterior costophrenic sinuses, thus suggesting middle mediastinal location.

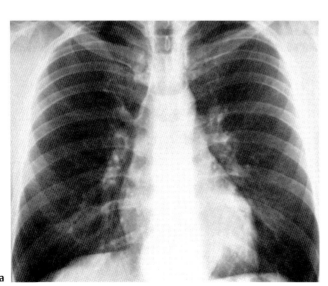
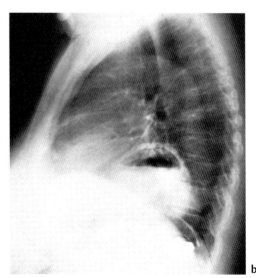

a                                    b

Fig. 2.**48 a, b    Hiatus hernia.** A retrocardiac mass with an air-fluid level.

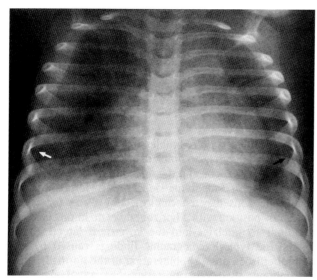

Fig. 3.**3   Bilateral pleural effusion** in a newborn (due to heart failure) as seen in supine position. There is a slight increase in the density of the right hemithorax, where the amount of fluid is greater and there is more replacement collapse of the lung, The layer of fluid in the pleural space is widest near the pulmonary apices. Major fissures are demonstrated because fluid enters into the lateral aspect of the fissures (arrows).

layer of fluid in the surrounding pleural space may be seen (Fig. 3.**3**).

Atypical distribution of pleural fluid may indicate localized parenchymal disease as well as pleural disease. In the region of parenchymal disease, the elastic recoil is decreased and fluid is attracted to those areas of the thorax where retraction force is greatest, e.g., where lung tissue is normal. Pleural fluid may simulate atelectasis or consolidation (Figs. 3.**4** and 3.**5**). Lateral decubitus view may help in visualizing the underlying parenchymal changes by redis-

tributing the fluid. Infrapulmonary (subpulmonary) pleural effusion (Fig. 3.**6**) without blunted costophrenic angles may represent a phenomenon of altered pulmonary recoil, but it is also seen with apparently normal lung. Although the lateral decubitus view is the best way of demonstrating an infrapulmonary fluid collection, it is important to know the following signs commonly present in erect films to raise suspicion of infrapulmonary effusion:

1. Infrapulmonary fluid is more common on the right; it can be bilateral.
2. In posteroanterior projection, the peak of the pseudodiaphragmatic configuration is lateral to that of the normal hemidiaphragm.
3. On the left side, there is an increased distance between the lung base and the gastric air bubble (this also occurs with gastric tumors and interposition of the liver or spleen) (Fig. 3.**6**). An indentation on the gastric air bubble represents the depressed diaphragm.
4. The posterior costophrenic gutter is usually blunted, although other signs of fluid in costophrenic angles are lacking.
5. In the lateral projection, the contour of the fluid is usually flattened anterior to the major fissure. This segment descends abruptly to the anterior costophrenic angle.
6. There may be a triangular mediastinal collection of fluid seen in the anteroposterior view.

Loculated or encysted pleural fluid may occur anywhere in the pleural space secondary to pleural adhesions. Samples of loculated pleural fluid are presented in Figures 3.**7** and 3.**8**. Encapsulated fluid in the lower half of the major fissure may mimic atelectasis and consolidation of the right middle lobe. However, encapsulated fluid does not obscure the minor fissure or right heart border as do atelectasis or consolidation of the middle lobe. Furthermore, encapsulated fluid has a spindle-shaped form, whereas the shadow of the diseased middle lobe has straight or slightly concave borders. Encapsulated fluid does not move in response to postural changes. Thus, encapsulated fluid and pleural thickening may have identical appearance.

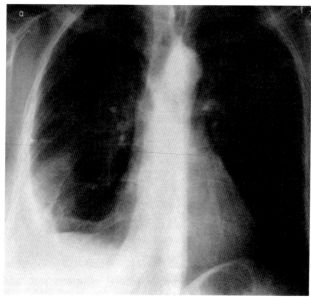

a

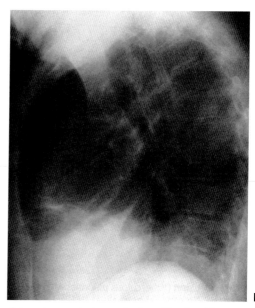

b

Fig. 3.**4 a, b   Right pleural effusion** (metastatic breast carcinoma, post left mastectomy) may mimic consolidation or atelecta-sis in anteroposterior projection. The densities are created by fluid in the fissures surrounding the middle lobe.

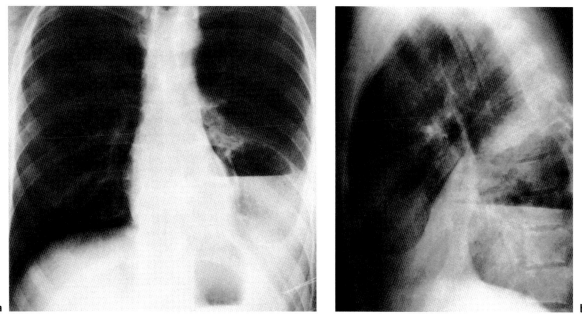

a                                                                                                    b

Fig. 3.**5 a, b**   **Atypical accumulation of pleural effusion** around a left lower lobe abscess containing an air-fluid level.

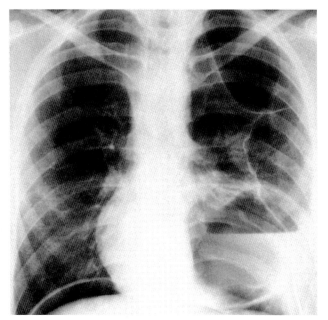

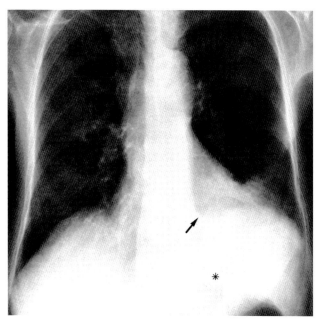

Fig. 3.**5 c**   **Post thoracentesis.** There is inadvertent pneumothorax and pneumoperitoneum. The fluid within the abscess remains, while the pleural collection has disappeared.

Fig. 3.**6**   **Infrapulmonary pleural effusion** on the left (chronic leukemia). The peak of the pseudodiaphragmatic configuration is more lateral than normal and there is increased distance between the lung base and the gastric air bubble (asterisk). A triangular rnediastinal collection of fluid is seen (arrow).

Pleural fluid tends to have an identical roentgenographic appearance independent of its nature (transudate, exudate, pus, blood). Transudate contains protein more than 30 g/l and exudate less than 30 g/l. Transudate is often present with heart or liver failure, nephrotic syndrome or Meigs syndrome. Infections, malignancies, collagen vascular diseases, etc often causes presence of exudate. Differential diagnosis of pleural fluid (effusion) therefore often has to be based on other radiographic manifestations of disease in the chest, patient history, and pleural tap.

Positive diagnosis is often, but not always, obtained from laboratory studies of the pleural fluid. In Table 3.**1**, emphasis has been put on associated radiologic findings as criteria for differential diagnosis.

Pleural effusion unassociated with other roentgenographic evidence of disease in the thorax is a nonspecific finding and the differential diagnosis depends on additional clinical information or roentgenographic findings elsewhere in the body.

Common causes of pleural fluid with the otherwise normal looking chest are:

1  infection of the pleura (*tuberculosis, viral diseases*) or of the abdomen (*pancreatitis, subphrenic abscess*);
2  extrathoracic carcinoma, either metastatic to the pleura or mediastinal nodes (most commonly due to *breast carcinoma*) or via diaphragmatic lymphatics (*carcinoma of the pancreas* or *retroperitoneal lymphoma*);
3  collagen diseases (*rheumatoid arthritis, systemic lupus erythematosus*);
4  *cirrhosis* with *ascites*;
5  closed *chest trauma* or *abdominal surgery*.

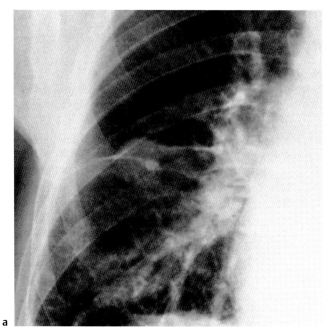

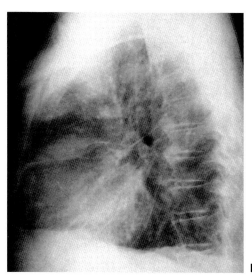

a

b

Fig. 3.**7 a, b**    **Encapsulated fluid in the minor fissure;** a pseudotumor, The lobulated effusion has a typical spindle-shaped form. Severe heart failure with interstitial pulmonary edema.

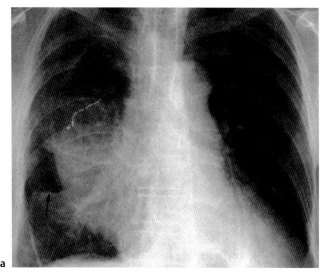

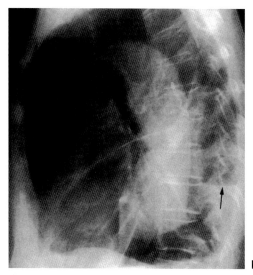

a

b

Fig. 3.**8 a, b    Loculated right posterior hydropneumothorax** post surgery for esophageal carcinoma. An air-fluid level is seen around the right lower lobe (arrows), secondary to the rupture of the displaced stomach which is seen as a density over the right heart border.

**Table 3.1   Differential Diagnosis of Pleural Effusion**

| Disease | Radiographic Findings | Comments |
|---|---|---|
| *Neoplasms* | | |
| Bronchogenic carcinoma | A common radiological manifestation of bronchial carcinoma at presentation is a pleural effusion. Obstructive pneumonitis associated with ipsilateral pleural effusion and eventual hilar or mediastinal lymphadenopathy. | The volume of effusion is usually large. Following aspiration it rapidly accumulates. It is commonly blood stained and contains malignant cells. |
| Lymphoma (Fig. 3.9) | Pleural effusion is associated with single or multiple areas of consolidation and hilar or mediastinal lymph node enlargement. Approximately one third of patients have pleural fluid. | Includes leukemia, Hodgkin's disease, and non-Hodgkin's lymphoma. Pleural effusion alone may occur especially in retroperitoneal lymphoma. |
| Metastatic neoplasm (Fig. 3.4) | Diffuse pulmonary densities and pleural effusion together with normal heart size. | Hematogeneous spread results generally in nodular densities. Lymphangitic spread results in linear densities (A and B lines) with eventual lymph node enlargement. Pleural effusion may be the only presenting finding. Breast cancer is the most common origin. Other primaries include pancreas, stomach, ovary and kidney. |
| Mesothelioma (Fig. 3.10) | Massive pleural effusion associated with nodular diffuse pleural thickening. Volume of ipsilateral hemithorax may be reduced despite massive opacification, | In the diffuse variety of mesothelioma, pleural effusion is a characteristic finding. History of asbestosis is common.<br>The local variety of mesothelioma presents as a peripheral mass and pleural effusion is rare. |
| Ovarian neoplasms (Meigs' syndrome) | Pleural fluid and/or ascites associated with benign ovarian tumour. | Pleural fluid and/or ascites secondary to ovarian neoplasms other than benign primary ovarian tumors or GI malignancies is called pseudo-Meigs' syndrome. |
| Carcinoma of pancreas | Effusion may occur by transport of fluid into thorax through diaphragmatic lymphatics, in such case pleural fluid is the only presenting sign in the chest roentgenogram. | Pleural fluid is negative for malignant cells unless metastatic deposits occur in pleura. |
| Multiple myeloma | Expanding soft-tissue lesion(s) arising from the chest wall is sometimes associated with pleural fluid. | Pleural effusion as a first sign of multiple myeloma is rare. |
| Primary neoplasms of the chest wall | May present an identical pattern compared to multiple myeloma. | Rare condition. Most are sarcomas. |
| *Infections* | | |
| Bacterial pneumonia | Variable findings including pleural effusions may be seen. Some more specific presentations are described below. | The pattern of pulmonary parenchymal disease is more diagnostic in pneumonia but not a specific finding. |
| Tularemia (*Francisella tularensis*) | Spherical or oval pulmonary densities. Enlarged lymph nodes and pleural effusion occurs in one third of patients. | Pleural effusions are more common in the typhoidal form (50–77%) than in the non-typhoidal form (8–26%). History of animal exposure is suggestive. Is a potential bioterrorism agent. |
| Q fever (*Coxiella burnetii*) | Q fever pneumonia has a nonspecific appearance on chest radiographs. A small pleural effusion may occur. | Zoonosis with a world wide distribution. Has caused epidemics in Eastern Europe. Is a potential bioterrorism agent. |
| *Staphylococcus aureus* | Pneumonia followed by empyema in infants and children is typical. Abscesses or pneumatoceles are common. | A confluent, destructive segmental pneumonia followed by empyema. Empyema occurs in 90% of cases in children and in 50% of adults. |
| Tuberculosis (Fig. 3.1) | Pleural effusion is often the only manifestation, associated parenchymal disease is rare. | A manifestation of primary tuberculosis more common in adults than in children. |
| *Clostridium perfringens* | A combination of pleural effusion, gas in soft tissues, and eventual segmental broncho-pneumonia. | Gas in soft tissues occurs more commonly in postoperative conditions or is associated with trauma. |
| Invasive fungal infections | A combination of cavitary pneumonia, pleural effusion (empyema), and chest wall involvement is highly suggestive of actinomycosis or nocardiosis. | Pleural effusion in other fungal infections of the chest is rare. Occasionally, (in 2%) histoplasmosis may present with pleural effusion indistinguishable from tuberculous pleuritis. Aspergillus may invade empyema cavity but is a rare cause of pleural effusion. |

*(continues on page 78)*

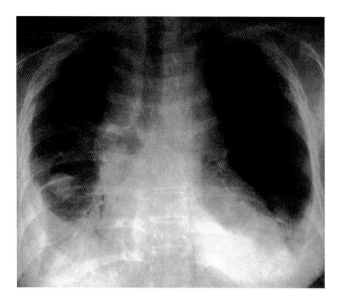

Fig. 3.**9** **Bilateral pleural effusion** in non-Hodgkin's lymphoma involving the mediastinum. Loculated fluid is seen in the minor fissure.

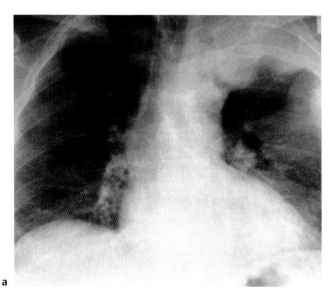

a

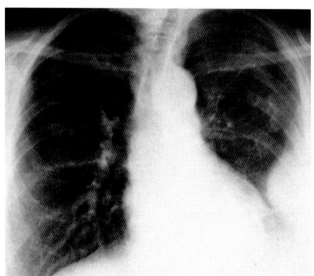

b

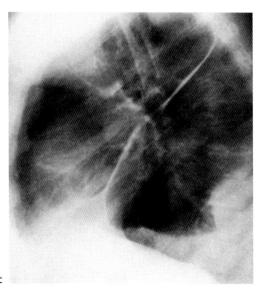

c

Fig. 3.**10 a-c** **Mesothelioma** (two cases), **a** A characteristic pattern of diffuse mesothelioma. Nodular thickening of pleura and pleural fluid are seen, **b, c** The tumor is seen as a local, slightly irregular, bulge in both AP and lateral projections, i.e., the tumor is more extensive than can be expected from a single view. Moderate amount of pleural fluid.

## Table 3.1   (Cont.) Differential Diagnosis of Pleural Effusion

| Disease | Radiographic Findings | Comments |
| --- | --- | --- |
| **Viral infections and** *Mycoplasma pneumoniae* | A combined interstitial and air-space pneumonia is a common presentation. Pleural effusion only is uncommon. | Occasionally, pleural effusion may be the only presenting sign. |
| **Amebiasis** *(Entamoeba histolytica)* | A rare combination of lower lobe consolidation, pleural effusion, and enlarged liver in a patient with diarrhea. | The organism may infiltrate from the liver abscess through diaphragm into pleura, lung and pericardium and cause this rare combination. |
| **Echinococcus (Hydatid disease)** | Hydropneumothorax occurs when an echinococcal cyst ruptures into the pleural space. | |
| **Abdominal inflammation** | Ipsilateral pleural effusion associated with evidence of abdominal disease. | Pleural effusion occurs commonly in pancreatitis (characteristically left-sided) and in subphrenic abscesses. |
| ***Miscellaneous*** | | |
| **Systemic lupus Erythematosus** | Bilateral pleural effusion, nonspecific cardiac enlargement, and basal atelectasis or pneumonia are suggestive. | Pulmonary changes are nonspecific. Cardiac enlargement is usually due to pericardial effusion. |
| **Rheumatoid arthritis** | A long-standing pleural effusion with or without pulmonary interstitial disease. | Pleural effusion may be the only presenting sign. The glucose content of the effusion is typically low. |
| **Wegener's granulomatosis** | A combination of pleural effusion and single or multiple pulmonary nodules, which may cavitate, associated with renal disease. | Effusion may be present in about half of the cases. |
| **Waldenstrom's macroglobulinemia** | Pleural effusion associated with diffuse reticulonodular pattern in the lungs. | Anemia, monoclonal IgM gammopathy, and lymphocytic or plasma cell infiltration of the bone marrow. Pleural effusion is present in roughly 50% of cases. |
| **Pulmonary embolism and infarction** (Fig. 3.11) | Variable patterns may include line shadows, segmental consolidation, elevation of the hemidiaphragm, small pleural effusions, and increased or decreased peripheral pulmonary vasculature. | Pleural effusion may occasionally be the only presenting sign. Pulmonary CT angiography is nowadays a common practice. Positive ventilation-perfusion scan is highly suggestive. |

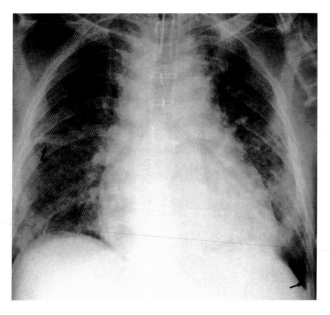

Fig. 3.**11**   **Pulmonary embolism.** Bilateral small pleural effusions (arrows), pulmonary edema pattern, and an enlarged heart are seen.

## Table 3.1    (Cont.) Differential Diagnosis of Pleural Effusion

| Disease | Radiographic Findings | Comments |
|---|---|---|
| **Congestive heart failure (Fig. 16.9)** | Cardiac enlargement associated with pleural effusion and clinical signs of cardiac decompensation, see Chapter 1 | Pleural effusion is right-sided or bilateral. |
| **Postmyocardial infarction syndrome** | See Chapter 1. Left-sided or bilateral pleural effusion is common (80%), often accompanied by pericardial effusion and/or pulmonary infiltrates. | Can occur a few days, or up to two months, after acute myocardial infarction. |
| **Constrictive pericarditis** | Signs of systemic venous hypertension associated with pericardial calcification (in about 50%) and pleural effusion (in about 50%). | |
| **Obstruction of superior vena cava or azygos vein** | Clinical signs of the superior vena cava syndrome, associated with mediastinal widening and pleural effusion. | May be caused by a tumor or, rarely, a benign process such as sclerosing mediastinitis. |
| **Asbestosis** | Three types of pleural changes occur alone or in combination with others: 1 Pleural plaques which calcify in about one third of cases; 2 pleural thickening and 3 pleural effusions. Associated pulmonary manifestations may produce a "shaggy heart" sign. | High incidence of associated bronchogenic carcinoma and mesolhelioma. |
| **Open or closed chest trauma (including surgery) (Fig. 3.8, Fig. 3.12)** | A wide variety of changes: fractured ribs, pulmonary hemorrhage or hematoma, mediastinal hematoma, aortic aneurysm, pneumothorax, pneumomediastinum. | The history or associated findings usually al-low a precise diagnosis. After abdominal surgery and closed chest trauma, pleural effusion may be the only presenting finding. |

*(continues on page 80)*

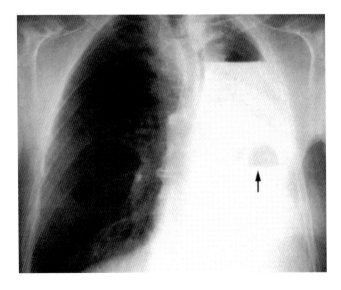

Fig. 3.**12  Surgical removal of the left lung.** There is gradual filling of the empty hemithorax with fluid. Displacement of the mediastinum to the left and of the gastric air bubble upwards (arrow) indicate passive accumulation of fluid into the left hemithorax. Active accumulation of fluid (such as metastatic) would displace neighbouring organs away from the fluid-filled hemithorax.

**Table 3.1 (Cont.) Differential Diagnosis of Pleural Effusion**

| Disease | Radiographic Findings | Comments |
|---|---|---|
| Chylothorax (Fig. 3.13) | After thoracic surgery and inadvertent injury to the thoracic duct, chylothorax (chylous effusion) may develop, often after a delay of a few days. | Chylous effusion may also be secondary to malignancy, parasites (filariasis) and lymphangiomyomatosis. |
| Sarcoidosis | Pleural effusion is rare (incidence 0.7 to 4%) in sarcoidosis and should be diagnosed only after exclusion of other more common causes of pleural effusion. | Miliary pulmonary shadows associated with pleural effusion is more likely due to disseminated metastases or tuberculosis. |
| Nephrotic syndrome Diminished plasma osmotic pressure | Commonly infrapulmonary effusion. | Biochemical assay of serum and urine shows proteinuria, hypoproteinemia and generalised edema. |
| Hydronephrosis | Pleural effusion without chest disease is a rare manifestation of hydronephrosis. | May be related to transport of fluid via diaphragmatic lymphatics. |
| Uremia, dialysis (Fig. 3.14) | Pleural effusion associated with pericardial effusion and/or pulmonary manifestations of uremia. | May mimic congestive heart failure. |
| Myxedema | Pleural effusion without distinctive features. | Pericardial effusion is more common. |
| Cirrhosis of the liver with ascites | Presents as pleural effusion without chest disease. | Ascites and other signs of cirrhosis are usually present. |
| Lymphedema | Pleural effusion associated with clinical findings of lymphedema. | Hypoplasia of the lymphatic system. |
| Familial Mediterranean fever (familial recurrent polyserositis) | Pleural effusion associated with osteoporosis, arthritis, and often pericarditis. | Hereditary, limited to Armenians, Arabs, and Sephardic (non-Ashkenazi) Jews. Typical manifestations include episodes of fever, with abdominal, thoracic or joint pain due to inflammation of the peritoneum, pleura, and synovial membrane. Amyloidosis may complicate the condition. |
| Drug-induced pleural effusion | Pleural effusion associated with interstitial lung disease or a lupus-like pattern. | Drugs: nitrofurantoin, hydralazine, procainamide. |

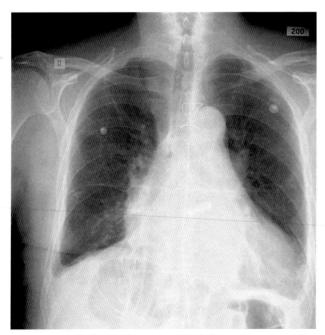

Fig. 3.**13** **Chylothorax** due to lacerated ductus thoracicus after thoracic aorta surgery in 70 years old male

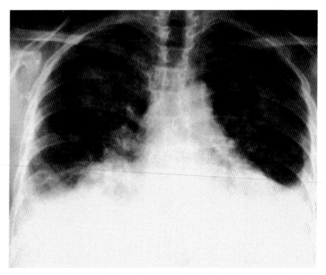

Fig. 3.**14** **Uremia.** Bilateral massive pleural effusions and patchy alveolar infiltrates (pulmonary edema).

## Table 3.2  Differential Diagnosis of Diaphragmatic Elevation

| Disease | Radiographic Findings | Comments |
|---|---|---|
| **Normal variation** | Usually right hemidiaphragm is 1–2,5 cm higher than left. Poor inspiration and obesity may cause apparent elevation. | In 10 % of population diaphragms are at the same level or left hemidiaphragm is higher than right. |
| **Eventration** | Abnormal elevation of all or a portion of an attenuated but otherwise intact diaphragmatic leaf. | More common on right side. Diaphragm muscle is permanently elevated, but retains its continuity. |
| **Phrenic nerve palsy (Fig. 3.15)** | The affected side does not move correctly. In inspirium affected side tends to rise instead of lowering. | May be due bronchogenic carcinoma, mediastinal metastasis, neurologic disease, injury to the phrenic nerve at any location. |
| **Pulmonary infarction secondary to pulmonary embolism. (Fig. 3.16)** | Chest X-ray signs are nonspecific. They may include subpleural consolidation, segmental collapse or plate atelectasis, pleural reaction with small effusion, elevation of hemidiaphragm of the affected side. Rarely cavitation of the infarct. | Patients with pulmonary embolic disease leads to infarction in about one third of cases. Pulmonary CT angiography is diagnostic. |

*(continues on page 82)*

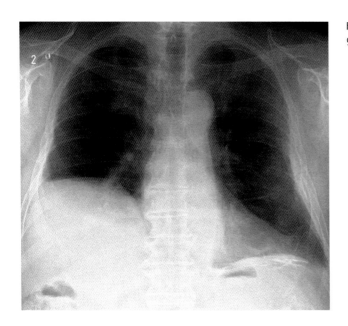

Fig. 3.**15**  **Phrenic nerve palsy.** The right hemidiaphragm is grossly elevated

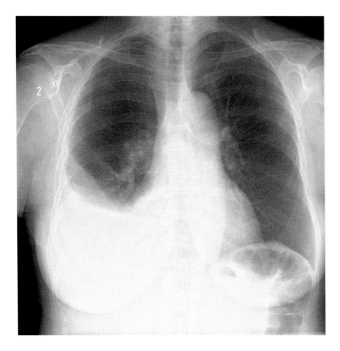

Fig. 3.**16**  **Pulmonary infarction.** Slightly elevated right hemidiaphragm, distorted branches of right lower lobe arteries and dilated main trunk of right pulmonary artery

**Table 3.2  (Cont.) Differential Diagnosis of Diaphragmatic Elevation**

| Disease | Radiographic Findings | Comments |
|---|---|---|
| **Pulmonary collapse because of bronchial obstruction (Fig. 3.17)** | Elevated hemidiaphragm. The cause of obstruction may not be seen. | Occlusion of a bronchus for any reason. |
| **Subphrenic inflammatory disease** | Elevated hemidiaphragm and restricted motion | Common causes:<br>*pancreatitis*<br>*subpherenic abscess*<br>*hepatic abscess*<br>*splenic abscess*<br>*cholecystitis*<br>*perforated ulcer* |
| **Increased abdominal volume (Fig. 3.18)** | Usually bilaterally elevated diaphragm | Common causes:<br>*ascites*<br>*pregnancy*<br>*hepatomegaly (splenomegaly)*<br>*large tumour*<br>*obesity* |
| **Old haemothorax<br>Old empyema<br>Post thoracotomy** | Decreased lung volume associated with pleural thickening | |
| **Post surgery** | Combination of pneumothorax and air fluid level. The volume of pneumothorax tends to decrease and eventually disappears | After pulmectomy or lobectomy the space fills with pleural fluid and hemidiaphragm raises. |
| **Diaphragmatic hernias** | May mimic unilateral diaphragmatic elevation | On lateral view Morgagni hernia is situated on the anterior portion and Bochdalek hernia on posterior location. |
| **Diaphragmatic trauma (Fig. 13.15)<br>Diaphragmatic splinting** | More commonly on the left side. | May mimic elevated diaphragm as soft tissues herniate into the hemithorax. Stomach and/or bowel herniates on the left and liver on the rigth side. |
| **Subpulmonic effusion (Fig. 3.6)** | This is not true elevation of diaphragm but pleural fluid collection between lung base and diaphragm. The distance between diaphragm and stomach air bubble is increased | Radiographic with horizontal X-rays on suspected side reveals fluid. |
| **Rib fracture** | Pain induced limited mobility of the diaphragm. | May be associated with hemo- or pneumothorax |

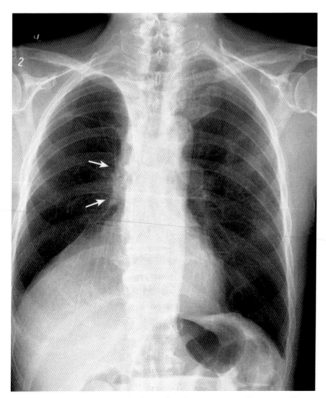

Fig. 3.**17**  Elevation of right hemidiaphragm secondary to **pulmonary collapse** (epidermoid carcinoma of right lower lobe bronchus)

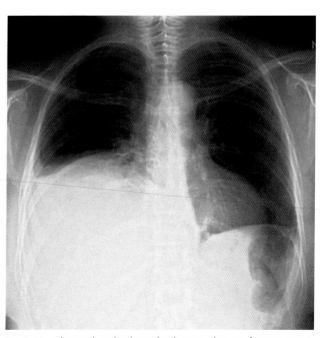

Fig. 3.**18**  Elevated right hemidiaphragm due to **breast carcinoma metastases to the liver**

# 4 Intrathoracic Calcifications

Calcifications in chest roentgenograms appear commonly. They are most frequently found in asymptomatic individuals as signs of "burned-out" disease or as the result of physiological calcification, such as calcification of the cartilagenous portions of the ribs or calcifications of the tracheobronchial tree. The causes of calcification of the soft tissues surrounding the thoracic cage are the same as those causing generalized calcification of periarticular soft tissues, and the reader should consult Chapter 7, Table 7.3.

Calcification of the aorta and other arteries is a common feature of old age in western countries and may have little diagnostic significance unless associated with other changes such as aneurysmatic dilatation of the artery. Atherosclerotic calcifications also commonly occur in the mitral and aortic annuli of the heart. Arteriosclerotic calcification of the coronary arteries is likewise common, but due to its high kVp, the routine chest radiograph rarely reveals such small calcifications in the heart or elsewhere. Multidetector CT is used for better visualization of cardiac calcifications. The lung is the most frequent visceral site of *metastatic calcifications*, which are most commonly associated with renal failure. Metastatic calcifications of the lungs are, however, rarely demonstrated radiographically. *Granulomatous calcifications* (Fig. 4.1) of the pulmonary parenchyma are common and diagnostically important, since demonstration of a calcified central nidus or laminated calcification in a pulmonary nodule is the most reliable sign of benignancy.

Diffuse or *miliary calcification* of the pulmonary parenchyma may be caused by several conditions but is less common than nodular calcification. Miliary calcifications of healed disseminated infections, mitral stenosis, or alveolar microlithiasis usually have distinctive features. *Calcification of pulmonary metastases* is uncommon. The most common primary neoplasm with calcified pulmonary metastases is osteosarcoma, but calcification may rarely occur in metastases of any mucinous adenocarcinoma. An eccentric calcification in a pulmonary mass can occasionally be found in a bronchogenic carcinoma engulfing a pre-existing granulomatous calcification.

Calcifications occur frequently in the thyroid, and may present as an upper mediastinal mass. Unfortunately, calcification of the thyroid mass is not a reliable sign of benignancy of the lesion. Other mediastinal tumors often have distinctive calcifications, e.g., demonstration of a bone or a tooth within a mass lesion is diagnostic for a *dermoid cyst*.

*Calcification of the pleura* may have the form of *continuous sheets* or *multiple calcified plaques*. The former type is usually unilateral and secondary to an old *pleural infection* (especially empyema or tuberculosis), or *hemothorax*. In such a case, calcium is usually deposited on the thickened visceral pleura and there is a thick layer of soft-tissue density between the calcification and the thoracic wall. Calcified or noncalcified plaques of the parietal pleura are typical of *asbestosis*, and the changes are usually bilateral. Associated pulmonary fibrosis is often lacking. If distinct calcification of apparently thickened pleura is lacking, nonpleural masses abutting the pleura should be considered. Such a finding may also be caused by intercostal fat or unusually prominent chest musculature. The latter is most common in the region from the 5th to 9th ribs in adults with inwardly concave lateral chest walls.

*Hilar calcifications* most commonly represent healed granulomatous infection of lymph nodes. They are usually stippled or amorphous and are irregularly distributed throughout the node. Ring calcification of the periphery of the lymph nodes (*"eggshell" calcification*) is unusual and characteristic of silicosis, but may very rarely also be found in sarcoidosis and in *irradiated Hodgkin's lymphoma*.

 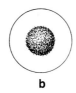  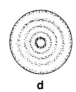 

a    b    c    d    e

Fig. 4.1 **Diagram of benign calcifications occurring in peripheral pul monary nodules: a** central nidus, **b** target lesion, **c** multiple punctate foci, **d** laminated, **e** conglomerate or "popcorn".

Types **a** and **c** occur in granulomas or hamartomas. Type **b** is characteristic of histoplasmosis. Type **d** occurs only in granulomas and type **e** is characteristic of hamartomas.

## Table 4.1 Differential Diagnosis of Cardiovascular Calcifications

| Location of the calcification | Causes or associated condition | Comments |
|---|---|---|
| **Aortic wall** (Figs. 4.2, 4.3) | Atherosclerosis Aneurysm Aortitis | Increased diameter of the aorta indicates an aneurysm. Increased distance between intimal calcification and the outer wall of the aorta suggests dissecting aneurysm. Heavy calcification of the dilated ascending aorta is characteristic of syphilitic aortitis. |
| **Sinus of Valsalva** (usually best seen in the lateral view) (Fig. 4.2) | Aneurysm of the sinus of Valsalva or, rarely, arteriosclerosis | Calcification may occur in the wall of the sinus and in the adjacent aorta. Heavy in syphilitic aneurysms. A thrombus in the aneurysm may calcify. |
| **Coronary arteries** (Fig. 4.4) | Arteriosclerosis of the coronary arteries (common) Coronary artery aneurysm (very rare) | The most common site of visible calcification is the proximal left circumflex artery. Easier to recognize in the lateral view as parallel linear or tubular calcifications. |
| **Aortic annulus or aortic valves** (Fig. 4.5) | Calcified annulus only: arteriosclerosis Valves with or without calcified annulus: Rheumatic aortic valve disease Arteriosclerosis Endocarditis Congenital defect of valve Hypercalcemia | Calcification of the annulus is usually heavy and distinct, whereas valvular calcifications are stippled and often superimposed by annulus, and not seen on plain films. If aortic valve disease appears before the age of 50 it is likely to be of rheumatic origin. |

*(continues on page 86)*

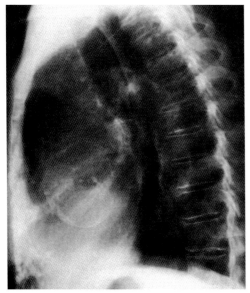

Fig. 4.**2**  **Calcified aneurysm** of the sinus of Valsalva. Widespread atherosclerotic calcification of the thoracic aorta, multiple calcified paratracheal lymph nodes and heavily calcified rib cartilages are present.

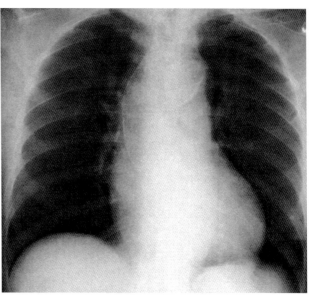

Fig. 4.**3**  **Syphilitic aortitis** with aneurysmal dilatation and heavy calcification of the ascending aorta.

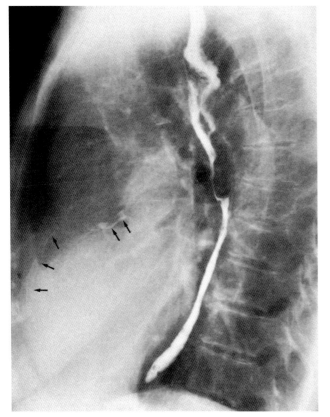

Fig. 4.**4**  **Coronary artery calcifications** (arrows).

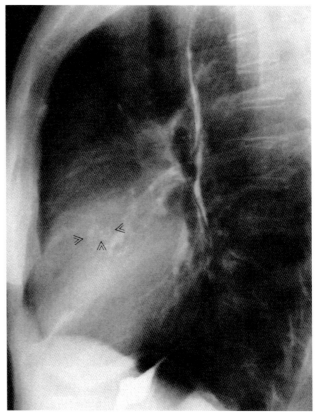

Fig. 4.**5**  **Aortic valve calcifications** (marked). Rheumatic stenosis and insufficiency of the aortic valve.

**Table 4.1   (Cont.) Differential Diagnosis of Cardiovascular Calcifications**

| Location of the calcification | Causes or associated condition | Comments |
|---|---|---|
| **Mitral annulus (Fig. 4.6)** | Arteriosclerosis | A dense curved or annular calcified band around the mitral valve. Usually insignificant, but rigid annulus may cause functional insufficiency of the mitral valve. |
| **Mitral valve** | Rheumatic mitral valve disease | Calcification may be indistinct and easily missed. The amount of calcification does not reflect the degree of functional disturbance. |
| **Myocardium (Fig. 4.7)** | Myocardial infarct Myocardial aneurysms due to infarct or rarely other causes such as syphilis Myocardial damage such as trauma, myocarditis, rheumatic fever (rare) Congenital (rare) Hyperparathyroidism (rare) Vitamin D overdosage (rare) | Calcification is usually smaller than the infarct. Most common at the apex with or without aneurysm. |
| **Left atrium (rare) (wall or intra-atrial)** | Rheumatoid mitral valve disease. Left atrial myxoma or thrombus | Calcification of the wall of the left atrium is seen as a thin, ring-like density in the frontal view. If the left atrial appendage is calcified, it is always due to a calcified thrombus. A calcified wall and a calcified thrombus may be difficult to differentiate from each other on the lateral view. |
| **Ductus arteriosus (rare)** | Patent ductus arteriosus | Difficult to differentiate from aortic calcification. May also occur with a closed ductus. |
| **Pericardium (Fig. 4.8)** | Pericarditis caused by: Tuberculosis Rheumatoid fever Bacterial pneumonia Myocardial infarction Viral infection Syphilis Histoplasmosis Asbestosis Trauma | The most common site of calcification is at the atrioventricular groove. Gross calcification of pericardium is associated with constrictive pericarditis in 50 % of cases. The so-called annular constrictive pericarditis (rigid atrioventricular groove) may mimic mitral valve disease. Extensive calcification of the circumflex coronary may mimic atrioventricular groove calcification. It may be difficult to differentiate between myocardial and pericardial calcifications. |

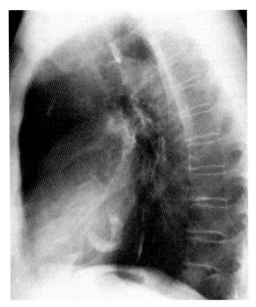

Fig. 4.**6**  **Calcified mitral annulus.**

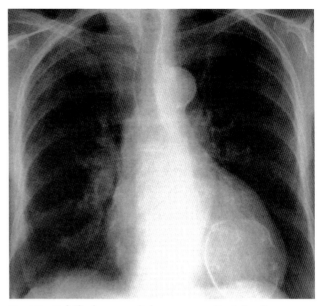

Fig. 4.**7**  **Calcified myocardial aneurysm** after infarction.

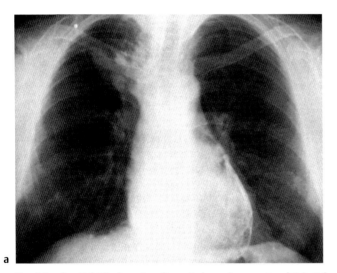

a

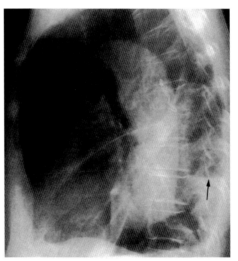

b

Fig. 4.**8 a, b**  **Calcified pericardium** (tuberculous pericarditis). Tuberculous granulomas and scarring in the right apex and an elevated right hilum are also evident.

**Table 4.2   Differential Diagnosis of Pulmonary Calcifications Solitary calcified pulmonary nodule of any size (single or occasionally multiple)**

| Causes or associated condition | Comments |
|---|---|
| Bronchogenic cyst (rare) | Two-thirds occur medially in the lungs, one-third in the mediastinum. Usually several centimeters wide, smooth, and well-defined. Rarely the thin cyst wall may calcify. Once infected, cyst may contain air. |
| Pulmonary arteriovenous fistula (rare) | Up to 6 cm slightly lobulated well-defined, multiple in one third of cases. Contains occasionally calcified phleboliths. Feeding artery and vein often identifiable. |
| Tuberculoma (common) (Fig. 4.9–4.10)<br>Histoplasmoma (common in endemic areas) (Fig. 4.11)<br>Coccidioidomycosis (rare) | A 0.5–5 cm round or oval lesion, with central calcification (calcific nidus, lamellated calcification or multiple punctate calcifications). A sizable target calcification is characteristic of histoplasmoma. A small lesion may be entirely calcified. Often associated with calcified regional lymph nodes and "satellite" lesions. May be multiple.<br>If the calcification is eccentric, bronchogenic carcinoma growing around a granuloma is a possibility. |
| Bronchial adenoma (rare) | Approximately 20–25 % of bronchial adenomas present as sharply circumscribed pulmonary nodules having a diameter of a few centimeters. Their calcification is rare. |
| Hamartoma (Fig. 4.12)<br>Chondroma (rare) | These constitute about 5 % of solitary peripheral nodules. Usually less than 4 cm in diameter and sharply marginated. "Popcorn" calcification of the cartilaginous portion is virtually diagnostic but calcification occurs in a minority of cases. May be multiple or grow slowly. |
| Hematogenous metastases (Fig. 4.13) | Calcification is rare; the most common primary tumor is an osteosarcoma. Rarely, a calcification is seen in pulmonary metastases of chondrosarcoma, synovial cell sarcoma, giant cell tumor of bone and mutinous carcinoma of colon, ovary, breast, thyroid, and (treated) choriocarcinoma. |
| Bronchopulmonary amyloidosis | A rare cause of usually multiple pulmonary nodules of variable size, which may show peripheral calcification or ossification. |
| Thrombus of pulmonary artery | Thrombi in the pulmonary arteries following embolism may rarely calcify. It is not associated with a mass lesion. |

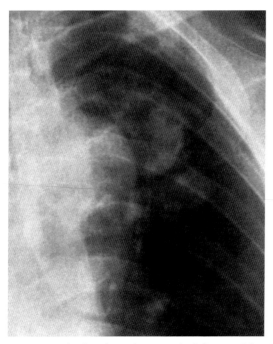

Fig. 4.**9** **Multiple tuberculomas** in the left upper lobe. Both central nidus and multiple punctate calcifications are seen.

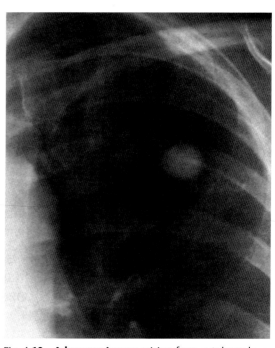

Fig. 4.**10** **Adenocarcinoma** arising from a tuberculous scar. The calcified nidus is eccentric.

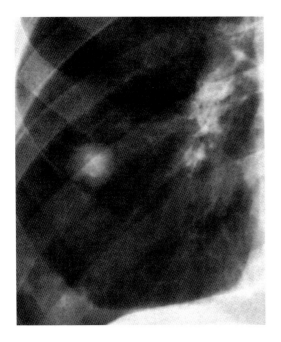

Fig. 4.**11**   **Histoplasmoma** with central target calcification.

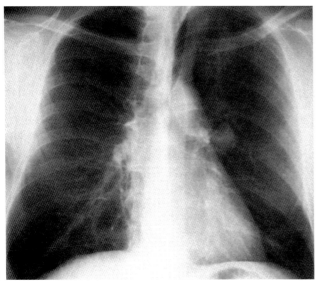

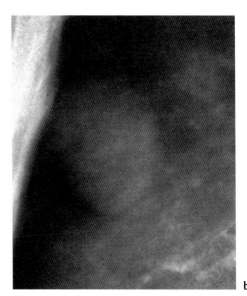

a                                                                                                                                                        b

Fig. 4.**12 a, b**   **Hamartoma.** A smooth 4-cm soft-tissue nodule with a faint conglomerate calcification in the center, better seen on the close-up lateral view (**b**).

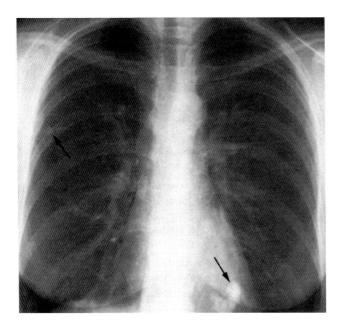

Fig. 4.**13**   **Calcified metastatic osteosarcoma.** One calcified lesion is seen in each lung (arrows).

**Table 4.3   Differential Diagnosis of Multiple Pulmonary Calcifications measuring less than 1 cm**

| Causes or associated condition | Comments |
|---|---|
| Histoplasmosis (healed) (Fig. 4.14) | Widespread densities of 3 to 4 mm in diameter throughout the lung fields containing punctate calcifications. Seen following disseminated histoplasmosis. Spleen may contain punctate calcifications, too. |
| Varicella (healed) (Fig. 4.15) | Miliary and larger densities with punctate calcifications a year or more after pulmonary chickenpox infection. |
| Mitral stenosis (Fig. 4.16) | Ossified and/or calcified nodules of up to 8 mm in diameter, predominantly in the right middle and lower lung fields. A rare but characteristic finding in mitral stenosis. |
| Pneumoconiosis due to inorganic dust, predominantly silicosis | Miliary and larger pulmonary densities, fairly sharply defined. May calcify. Hilar (eggshell) calcification may be present, too. |
| Alveolar microlithiasis (Fig. 4.17) | Extremely sharply defined, less than 1 mm, sandlike densities diffusely involving both lungs with an overall greater density in the lower than upper zones are diagnostic. |
| Metabolic or metastatic calcification (primary or secondary hyperparathyroidism, hypervitaminosis D, milk alkali syndrome, intravenous calcium therapy) | A very rare cause of alveolar calcification that mimics alveolar disease. Calcium may precipitate, especially at sites of pneumonic exudation. May occur within 3 weeks of open-heart surgery in children, and slowly regress. |

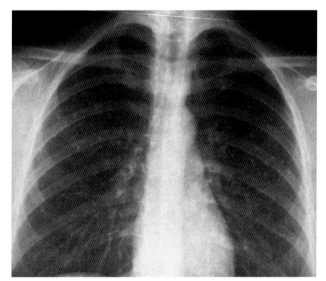

Fig. 4.**14   Healed disseminated histoplasmosis.** Miliary calcifications.

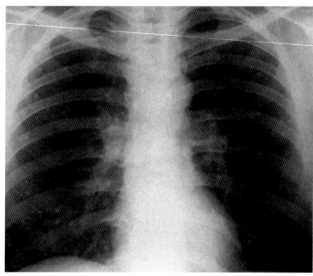

Fig. 4.**15   Healed varicella pneumonia.** Miliary and larger densities with punctate calcifications.

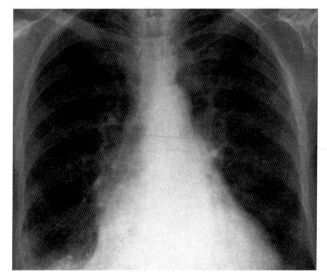

Fig. 4.**16   Mitral stenosis** with pulmonary ossification, best seen in the right lower lung field.

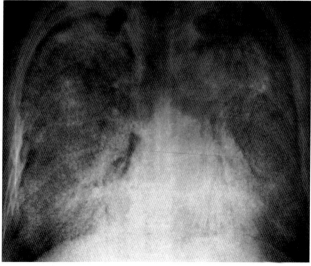

Fig. 4.**17   Alveolar microlithiasis.** Sand-like, sharp densities are seen throughout the lungs, primarily in the lower lobes. Apices show pleural thickening, bullous cavities and scarring consistent with old tuberculosis.

## Table 4.4    Differential Diagnosis of Pleural Calcifications

| Causes or associated condition | Comments |
| --- | --- |
| **Residue of**<br>  hemothorax<br>  pyothorax<br>  tuberculous pleuritis (Fig. 4.18) | Calcification and thickening of the visceral pleura or discrete plaques in the lower and middle fields. A thick layer of soft-tissue density is interposed between the calcific layer and the thoracic wall. Usually unilateral. |
| **Asbestosis (Fig. 4.19)**<br>talcosis | Pleural plaques and thickening originate from the parietal pleura. Usually bilateral and commonly diaphragmatic in position. Pulmonary parenchymal changes may be absent. Pleural calcifications are present in less than 50 % of cases. |

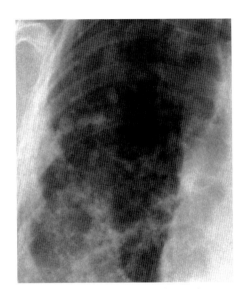

Fig. 4.**18**  **Residue of tuberculous pleuritis.** Vertical sheet-like calcifications and discrete plaques are seen on the right side. A layer of soft tissue between the calcification and thoracic wall is seen laterally.

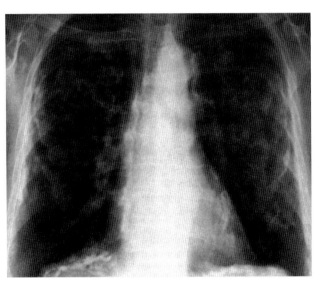

Fig. 4.**19**  **Asbestosis.** Bilateral pleural plaques and calcifications are seen along the chest wall, diaphragm and mediastinum. Calcifications tend to follow the course of the ribs. Parenchymal changes are not prominent.

**Table 4.5   Differential Diagnosis of Hilar or Mediastinal Calcifications**

| Causes or associated condition | Comments |
| --- | --- |
| **Thyroid mass** | Most commonly seen in the upper anterior mediastinum or less frequently in the upper posterior mediastinum. Calcification within the mass is frequent. Calcification occurs in both benign and malignant masses. |
| **Dermoid tumors**<br>**Teratoma (Fig. 4.20)**<br>**Thymoma**<br>**Neurogenic tumors (neurilemoma, neurofi-broma, gan-glioneuroma, neuroblastoma, paraganglioma)** | Calcification may be present around the lesion, particularly of dermoid cysts, but it has little differential diagnostic value. If bone is demonstrated within the lesion, the diagnosis of dermoid cyst is made with certainty. Neurogenic tumors may contain speckled calcification and are usually seen in the posterior mediastinum. If rib destruction is associated in a child, neuroblastoma is likely. |
| **Radiation therapy (Fig. 4.21, 4.22)** | Lymph node calcification in the mediastinum occurs after radiation therapy of mediastinal lymphoma or metastases, and rarely after chemotherapy. |
| **Tuberculosis**<br>**Histoplasmosis (Fig. 4.23)** | Amorphous or irregular calcification of involved nodes. Often associated with the Ghon lesion (parenchymal scar with calcification). |
| **Granulomatous mediastinitis**<br>**Sclerosing mediastinitis**<br>**(Idiopathic mediastinal fibrosis)** | Associated with tuberculosis or histoplasmosis, rarely silicosis or nocardiosis (granulomatous) or idiopathic. Mediastinal widening appears dense due to fine diffuse calcification that may be present even in absence of calcifications in plain films. |
| **Silicosis (Fig. 4.24)**<br>**sarcoidosis (rarely) (Fig. 4.25)**<br>**coccidioidomycosis (very rarely)** | Ring calcification of the periphery of lymph nodes, usually affecting bronchopulmonary lymph nodes. |
| **Calcified tracheal cartilage (Fig. 4.26)** | A common finding in elderly patients; no diagnostic significance. |

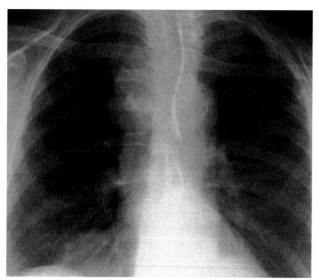

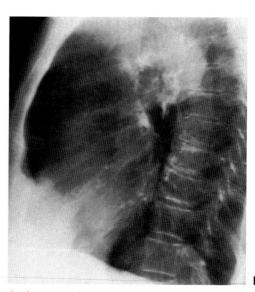

a  b

Fig. 4.**20 a, b   Upper middle mediastinal teratoma** containing characteristic calcified structures. The patient also has an anterior diaphragmatic hernia on the right side and a posterior diaphragmatic hernia on the left side.

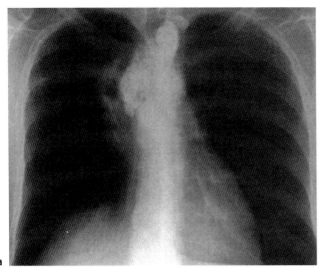

a

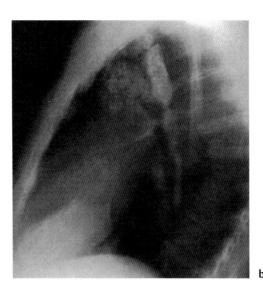

b

Fig. 4.**21 a, b   Calcified enlarged lymph nodes** after irradiation of Hodgkin's disease.

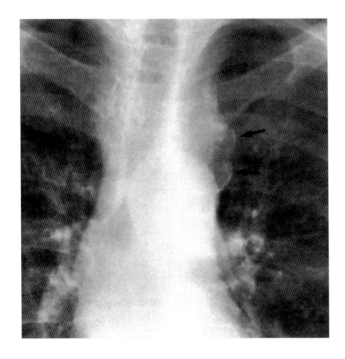

Fig. 4.**22   Eggshell calcifications** after irradiation of mediastinal metastases of seminoma are seen on the left, above the aortic knob.

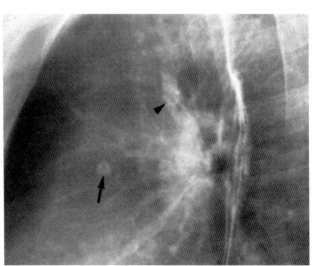

a

b

Fig. 4.**23 a, b   Calcified Ghon complex.** Laminated calcification of a granuloma in the anterior segment of the right upper lobe

(arrow) and amorphous calcification of a lymph node above the right hilum (arrowhead).

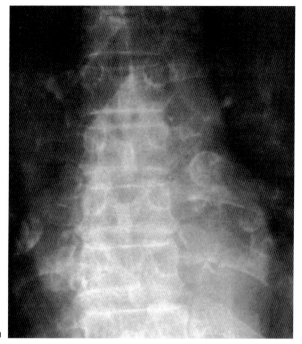
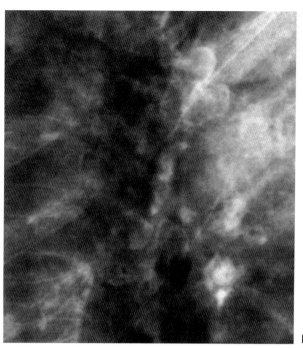

Fig. 4.**24 a, b    Silicosis.** Hilar lymph nodes contain characteristic "egg-shell" calcifications.

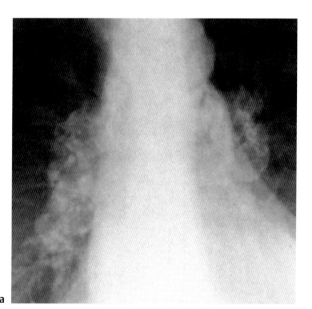
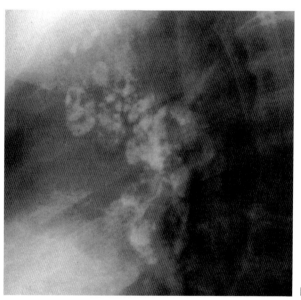

Fig. 4.**25 a, b    Sarcoidosis.** Enlarged hilar and mediastinal lymph nodes are extensively calcified, some of them showing the egg-shell pattern. A rare finding in sarcoidosis.

Fig. 4.**26    Extensive calcification of cartilaginous rings of the trachea and bronchi.** Granulomatous calcification of a subcarinal lymph node is also seen. Age 81.

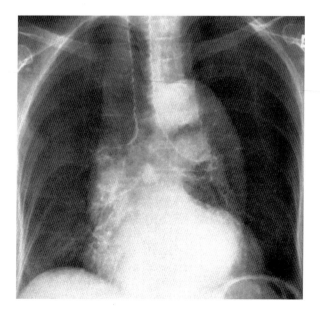

# 5 Alveolar Infiltrates and Atelectasis

An increase in the radiologic density of the lung may be caused by a pulmonary or an extrapulmonary process. Differentiation between these two entities should be attempted first whenever an increased density is observed in the lung (Figs. 5.1–5.3).

*Normal* and *pathologic structures of the chest wall* can cause an opacification in a lung field and simulate at times pulmonary disease. In women, the density of the lower lung fields is altered on the frontal examination by the presence and size of the breasts. Similarly, the pectoralis muscle, particularly when strongly developed, or an overlying scapula

may produce a localized increase in lung density. Whereas the recognition of normal soft tissue and bony structures does not usually cause any difficulty because of their constant anatomic location, a pathologic condition such as a tumor or a hematoma of the chest wall is more likely to be confused with a pulmonary process. Radiographic evaluation in two projections and/or clinical examination of the patient should, however, allow easy differentiation between a chest wall and a pulmonary lesion.

A unilateral increase in lung density is found when the frontal chest radiograph is taken in a slightly *rotated position*.

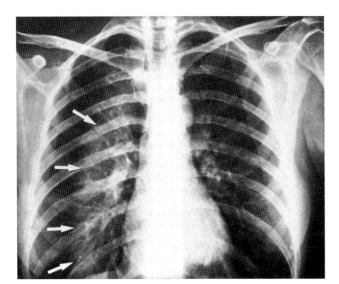

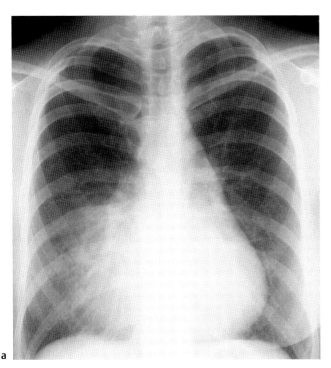

Fig. 5.1  Artifact caused by long hair combed in a ponytail simulating an infiltrate in right lung (arrows).

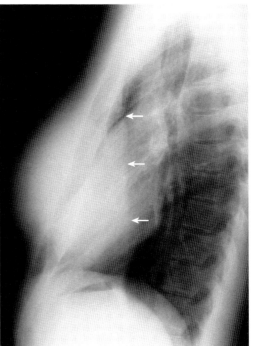

Fig. 5.**2 a, b  Pectus excavatum deformity.** A large opacity is evident in the lower portion of the right hemithorax contiguous with the thoracic spine mimicking a right middle lobe infiltrate (**a**). This is however a normal finding in patients with severe pectus deformity (**b**) caused by the posteriorly displaced sternum (arrows) resulting in compression of the adjacent right lung parenchyma and displacement of the heart towards the left.
▽

a

b

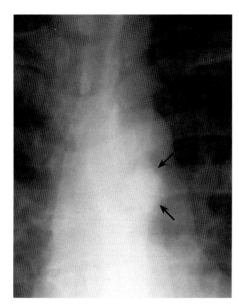

Fig. 5.**3**  **Osteophytosis in a costovertebral joint.** A round opacity (arrows) is overlying the left seventh rib posteriorly in the area of the costovertebral joint caused by advanced degenerative changes including marked hyperostosis in this articulation that could be mistaken for either a pulmonary or calcified mediastinal lesion.

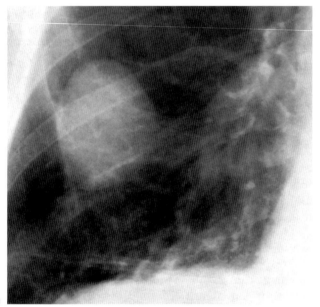

a

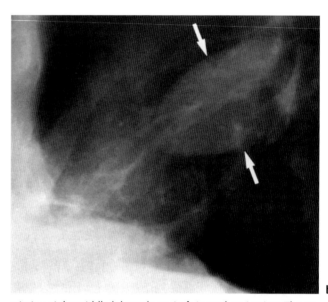

b

Fig. 5.**4**  **Loculated pleural effusion in major fissure** (lower half). **a** Anteroposterior projection: A homogeneous and well defined density projects into the right lower lung field. Smaller (thinner) fluid accumulations in that location are usually poorly defined and may mimic a right middle lobeatelectasis. **b** Lateral projection: The encapsulated fluid accumulation is spindle-shaped, with characteristically convex borders (arrows). Its long axis parallels the major fissure, which can often be seen exiting the density at one or both poles.

The lung, on which the spine is superimposed because of the rotation, usually demonstrates an increase in density. This is produced by the musculature around the spine that absorbs a significant portion of the roentgen beam passing through. A similar effect may also be found by incorrect centering of the roentgen beam or in patients with scoliosis. It is easy to recognize when the chest radiograph is centered off midline, as there is a variable distance between the lateral chest walls and the film margins: the side more distant from the midline is less exposed and appears lighter. On a supine chest film a pleural effusion layering out posteriorly may also mimic a unilateral underexposed (light) film.

Common causes for a bilateral and symmetrical increase in lung density of a healthy person are poor inspiration and underexposure of the film.

*Pleural abnormalities* may occasionally be difficult to differentiate from pulmonary lesions. A loculated effusion in the minor fissure could be mistaken for a neoplasm, although its location and radiographic appearance (a sharply demarcated and spindle-shaped lesion in both frontal and lateral projection) are quite characteristic. Furthermore the extremities of the loculated interlobar effusion blend imperceptibly with the interlobar fissure when viewed tangentially. Loculated fluid accumulation in the lower half of the major fissure is occasionally difficult to differentiate from a *right middle lobe atelectasis*. The encapsulated fluid has convex borders in the lateral projection and does not obscure the right heart border in the anteroposterior projection (Fig. 5.**4**). Furthermore, the minor fissure may be visible as a separate entity in one or both projections.

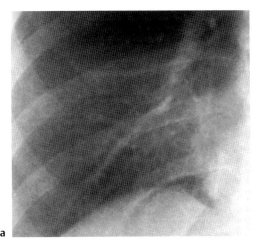
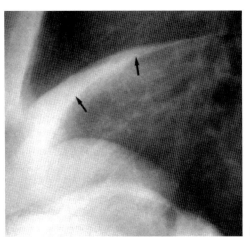

Fig. 5.**5**  **Right middle lobe atelectasis. a** Anteroposterior projection: A poorly defined pulmonary density obliterates the adjacent right heart border (positive "silhouette sign"; see Fig. 5.**8**, for negative "silhouette sign" with right lower lobe atelectasis). **b** Lateral projection: A well defined triangular density with characteristic concave inferior border (arrows) is evident. Furthermore, the minor fissure cannot be seen in either projection as a separate shadow, since this fissure constitutes the superior border of the triangular density.

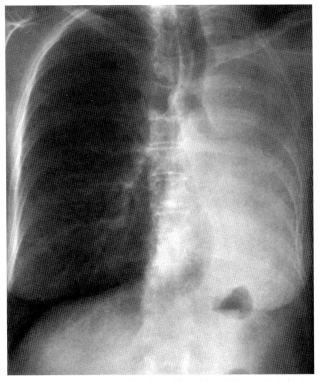
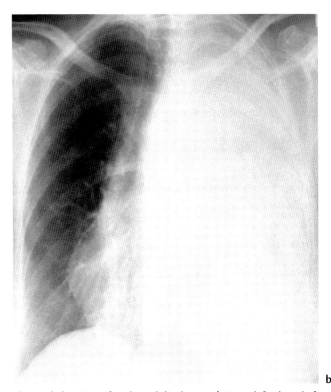

Fig. 5.**6**  **Complete opacification of one hemithorax (atelectasis versus pleural effusion). a** Total atelectasis of the left lung caused by bronchogenic carcinoma. Opacification of the left hemithorax is associated with signs of loss of volume: shifting heart and mediastinum toward the atelectasis, approximation of ribs, and elevation of ipsilateral diaphragm. **b** Large left pleural effusion caused by ovarian carcinoma. Opacification of the left hemithorax is associated with signs of mass effect: shifting of heart and mediastinum away from the pleural effusion and depresston of the ipsilateral diaphragm.

An atelectasis involving the entire right middle lobe has straight or concave margins in the lateral projection, and tends to obliterate the adjacent right heart border (positive "silhouette sign") in the anteroposterior projection (Fig. 5.**5**). The minor fissure is never seen as a separate linear density.In the upper half of the major fissure, an encapsulated fluid accumulation may, particularly on the frontal view, be confused with a pulmonary mass. On the lateral view, however, the encapsulated fluid has a characteristic elliptical shape with the long axis of the density paralleling the course of the major fissure. The encapsulated fluid blends at both ends with the fissure, provided the latter is visible. An infrapulmonary effusion may atypically extend into the posteromedial gutter, simulating a *lower lobe atelectasis.*

Opacification of a hemithorax by either massive atelectasis or effusion should not be difficult to differentiate, since the former is associated with radiographic signs of loss of volume (e.g., shifting of the heart and mediastinum toward the atelectasis, approximation of ribs, and elevation of the ipsilateral hemidiaphragm), where as the latter is an expanding process displacing the adjacent organs away from the effusion (Fig. 5.**6**). Complete Opacification of a hemi-

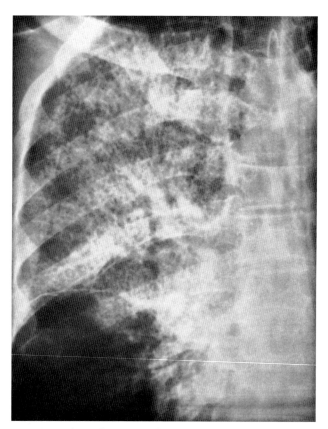

Fig. 5.**7** **Air bronchogram** in the right upper lobe. Air containing bronchi are visible, since they are surrounded by an alveolar infiltrate caused by pneumococcal pneumonia.

thorax with signs of volume loss similar to an atelectasis is also found after *pneumonectomy*.

In *alveolar lung disease* as defined in this chapter, the air in the alveolar and peripheral airways is replaced by fluid or tissue, resulting radiographically in opacities ranging in size from a few millimeters to several centimeters. Alveolar infiltrates may involve a segment or even a whole lobe, in which case boundaries of the resulting parenchymal consolidation are sharply demarcated. On the other hand, a large number of superimposed and partly confluent alveolar infiltrates may produce nonhomogeneous and rather poorly defined lung densities.

*Air bronchograms* are commonly found in alveolar lung disease, where the air-containing bronchi become clearly visible because of the surrounding infiltrates (Fig. 5.7). However, an air bronchogram is not diagnostic of alveolar disease, since an increase in the density of the peribronchial tissue is occasionally caused by interstitial or atelectatic lung disease. Whereas the absence of an air bronchogram in a lung density does not rule out alveolar disease, its presence is diagnostic for lung parenchyma involvement as opposed to pleural or extrapleural disease. The radiographic demonstration of an air bronchogram leads strongly away from a diagnosis of a malignant pulmonary neoplasm, with the exceptions of alveolar cell carcinoma and lymphoma. Air in the lung can be replaced by either fluid, cells, or solid substances under the following conditions: 1 the osmotic pressure of the blood is too low (e.g., hypoproteinemia); 2 the blood pressure in the capillaries is too high (e.g., heart failure); 3 the capillary permeability is increased (e.g., inhalation of noxious gases); 4 the barrier between blood and air space is defective (e.g., bleeding); 5 liquid or solid materials are aspirated; 6 abnormal material is secreted (e.g., cystic fibrosis) or deposited (e.g., alveolar proteinosis); and 7 cells are growing (e.g., neoplasm) or invading (e.g., infection and inflammation) the air space. In an atelectasis the resorbed air is not replaced by any material. All the aforementioned conditions may radiographically produce opacities within the lung parenchyma and their differentiation depends on size, location, and distribution, the association of other radiographic findings, and knowledge of the patient's clinical history and physical examination. The differential diagnosis of alveolar infiltrates and atelectasis is discussed in Table 5.**1**.

## Table 5.1  Alveolar Infiltrates and Atelectasis

| Disease | Radiographic Appearance | Comments |
|---|---|---|
| Bronchial adenoma (Fig. 5.8) | Centrally located tumors arising from major bronchi (80%) often present as recurrent segmental and lobar atelectasis and/or obstructive pneumonia.<br>Pulmonary, hilar and bony metastases (lytic and blastic) occur occasionally with carcinoids. | 90% in patients between 30 and 50 years old. Slightly more common in females. Histologically 3 types: 1 carcinoid adenomas (90%) including oncocytoid type; 2 cylindromas (7%) and 3 mucoepidermoid tumors (3%). |
| Papillomas and other benign endobronchial tumors | Atelectasis and obstructive pneumonia | Rare. Papillomas may originate in larynx or trachea. They may be multiple and commonly occur in children. |
| Bronchogenic carcinoma (Fig. 5.9) | Persistent atelectasis and obstructive pneumonia (usually segmental, but may also be lobar or, less commonly, involve a whole lung) is most common radiologic presentation.<br>Ipsilateral hilar enlargment and when further advanced, mediastinal widening is often associated with the parenchymal disease. Pleural effusions are simultaneously present in approximately 10% of all cases.<br>*Pancoast* or *superior pulmonary sulcus tumors* present as unilateral apical mass, often with destruction of the adjacent rib. | Approximately 75% occur in males in their 5th and 6th decades.<br>Inhalation of carcinogens (cigarette smoke, asbestos, etc.) are predisposing factors. Incidence in cigarette smokers ten times higher than in nonsmokers. Carcinomas also originate in tuberculous scars with higher than purely coincidental incidence.<br>Histologically adenocarcinomas (50%), squamous cell carcinomas (30%), small cell carcinomas (15%) and large cell carcinomas (5%) are distinguished. Pancoast tumors often present clinically with Horner's syndrome. |

*(continues on page 100)*

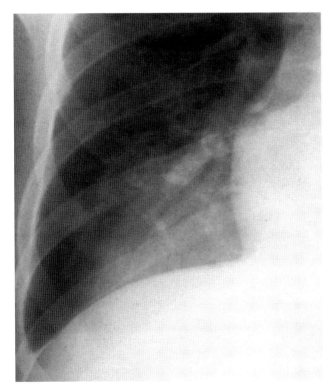

Fig. 5.**8**  **Bronchial adenoma** (carcinoid type) causing right lower lobe atelectasis. Note that the right cardiac border is not obliterated by the atelectatic right lower lobe, since these anatomical structures are not contiguous (negative "silhouette sign").

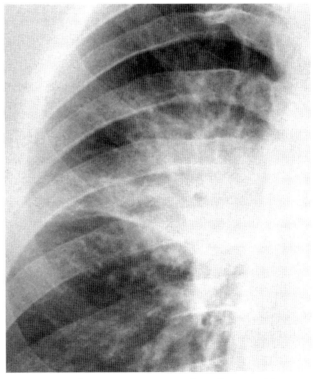

Fig. 5.**9**  **Bronchogenic carcinoma** in the right upper lobe causing obstructive pneumonitis.

**Table 5.1   (Cont.) Alveolar Infiltrates and Atelectasis**

| Disease | Radiographic Appearance | Comments |
|---|---|---|
| Bronchioloalveolar carcinoma (alveolar cell carcinoma) (Fig. 5.10) | Peripheral homogeneous consolidation ranging in size from 1 cm in diameter to the involvement of an entire lobe. Air bronchograms are often present. Diffuse bilateral involvement with fluffy confluent infiltrates occurs in a more advanced stage. Hilar enlargement and pleural effusions are occasionally associated with the pulmonary involvement. | Most commonly found in middle-aged patients, without sex predilection. |
| Lymphoma (Fig. 5.11) | Perihilar infiltrate is the most common parenchymal manifestation. Peripheral consolidations and atelectasis secondary to endobronchial lymphoma are less common. Air bronchograms are often encountered. Hilar and/or mediastinal involvement is usually present with lung parenchyma involvement. | Primary pulmonary lymphoma is rare and radiographically indistinguishable from *pseudolymphoma*, a rare benign condition not associated with hilar or mediastinal adenopathy. Any alveolar lung infiltrate in a patient with known lymphoma is more likely to represent an infectious than a lymphomatous process. |
| Kaposi's sarcoma (Fig. 5.12) | Bilateral, symmetric, poorly defined nodular opacities are characteristic. Nodules measure up to 3 cm and tend to coalesce. Pleural effusions (50%) and hilar or mediastinal adenopathy (10%) may be associated. | Occurs almost exclusively in HIV-infected male homosexuals and rarely in other HIV-infected patients. |
| Amyloidosis (tracheobronchial form) | Endobronchial amyloid deposition may cause atelectasis and obstructive pneumonia involving a segment to an entire lung. | Pulmonary manifestations occur in primary amyloidosis or in conjunction with multiple myeloma. |
| Arteriovenous malformation | Homogeneous, sharply defined and often somewhat lobulated density with lower lobe predilection. Identification of feeding and draining vessel not always possible. Multiple lesions in approximately one-third of patients. | Approximately half of the patients have arteriovenous fistulas elsewhere (*hereditary hemorrhagic telangiectasia* or *Rendu-Osler-Weber's disease*). |
| *Pneumonia, bacterial* | | |
| Staphylococcus aureus (Fig. 5.13) | Patchy consolidations without air bronchograms characteristic. Bilateral in over 60%. Both pneumatocele and abscess formations occur frequently and may contain air-fluid levels. Pneumatoceles have characteristically thin walls that differentiate them from abscesses. Pleural effusion (or empyema) is found in 50% of adults and is even more common in children. | Common in hospital patients and compromised hosts. Pneumatoceles are cyst-like lesions resulting from a check-valve-obstructed communication with a bronchus. They are particularly common in children. |
| Streptococcus pyogenes | Similar to staphylococcal pneumonia: patchy or homogeneous consolidations without air bronchograms and a high incidence of accompanying pleural effusion. Differentiating features are a lower tendency to form abscesses and pneumatoceles. | Streptococcal pneumonias are often found in mixed or secondary infections. |

*(continues on page 102)*

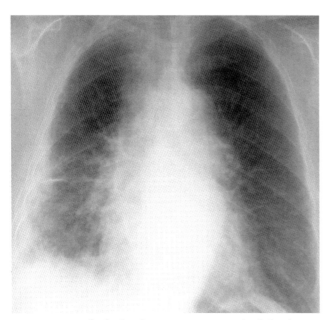

Fig. 5.**10  Bronchioloalveolar carcinoma.** Poorly defined, confluent nodular opacities are seen in the right lower lobe. A small right pleural effusion is also present. Furthermore smaller, poorly defined nodules are scattered throughout the remaining right lung and left lower lung zone.

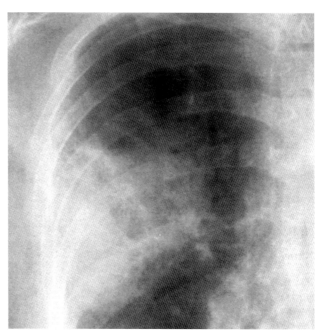

Fig. 5.**11  Non-Hodgkin lymphoma.** A large consolidation is seen in the right upper lobe.

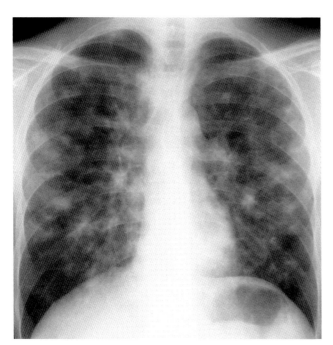

Fig. 5.**12  Kaposi's sarcoma.** Bilateral, symmetric, poorly defined, partly coalescent nodules are seen.

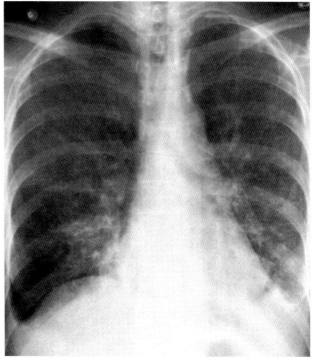

Fig. 5.**13  Staphylococcal pneumonia** presenting as bilateral patchy infiltrates in the lower lobes with small pleural effusions.

**Table 5.1   (Cont.) Alveolar Infiltrates and Atelectasis**

| Disease | Radiographic Appearance | Comments |
|---|---|---|
| **Pneumonia, bacterial (cont.)** | | |
| **Pneumococcus (Streptococcus pneumoniae) (Fig. 5.14)** | Homogeneous consolidation with air bronchograms characteristic. Usually confined to one lobe. Another presentation observed with apparently increasing frequency consists of patchy bronchopneumonia-like infiltrates that may be bilateral. Small pleural reactions occur in 20% of cases. Cavitation is rare. | Common in alcoholics and compromised hosts, but also occurs in otherwise healthy people. In children, the disease may present as a spherical, well-circumscribed pulmonary density. |
| **Klebsiella (Fig. 5.15)** | Large well-defined homogeneous consolidation with air bronchograms similar to pneumococcal pneumonia. Differentiating features from the latter are: 1 upper lobe predilection, 2 tendency to expand involved lobe, 3 abscess formation and pleural effusion common. | Common in alcoholics and in elderly patients with chronic pulmonary disease. |
| **Legionella (Fig. 5.16)** | Poorly defined round or diffuse infiltrates central or peripheral in location, usually beginning in one lobe and spreading in two-thirds of cases to the other lung. Pleural effusion may be present. Cavitation and hilar adenopathy does not occur. | Legionnaires' disease is an acute Gram-negative bacterial pneumonia found in local outbreaks or as sporadic cases. Clearing of pneumonic infiltrates within one month. |
| **Pseudomonas (Fig. 5.17)** | Bilateral patchy infiltrates with predilection for the lower lobes, progressing rapidly to extensive homogeneous consolidations with air bronchograms, are characteristic. Abscess formation is common. Small but radiographically not very conspicuous effusions are usually present. | Almost invariably in compromised hosts who acquire the disease in the hospital. Organism resistant to almost all antibiotics. |
| **Haemophilus influenzae (Fig. 5.18)** | Patchy, poorly defined infiltrates, predominantly in the lower lobes, unilateral or bilateral. Pleural effusions occur frequently and may be the dominant feature, especially in children. | Most common organism cultured from purulent expectorations of patients with chronic pulmonary disease, although its pathogenicity is still in doubt, since it is also commonly found in the flora of healthy people. |

*(continues on page 104)*

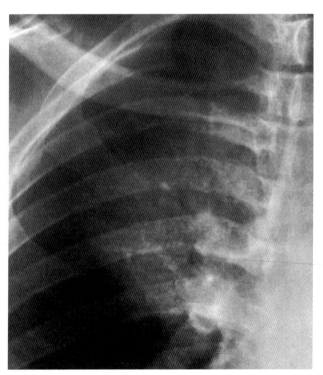

Fig. 5.**14** **Pneumococcal pneumonia** presenting as consolidation with air bronchogram in the anterior segment of the right upper lobe. The pneumonic process obliterates the lateral border of the adjacent ascending aorta (positive "silhouette sign"). See also Fig. 5.**5**.

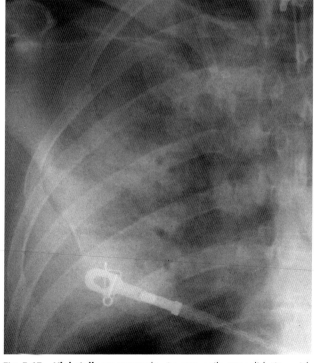

Fig. 5.**15** **Klebsiella pneumonia.** An expansile consolidation with air bronchograms is involving the entire right upper lobe.

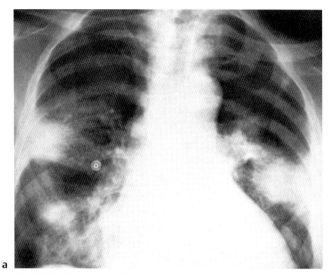

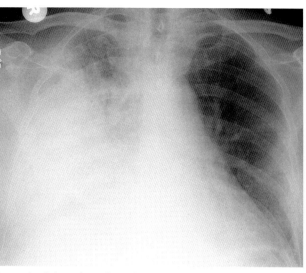

a

b

Fig. 5.**16 a, b   Legionella pneumonia (Legionnaires' disease)** (2 cases). **a** Bilateral poorly defined, peripheral infiltrates are seen.

**b** Besides bilateral small patchy infiltrates a large consolidation is seen in the right lung.

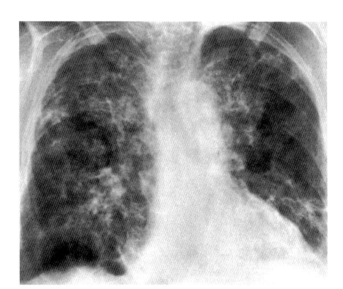

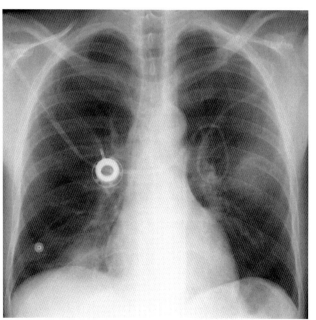

Fig. 5.**17    Pseudomonas pneumonia.** Extensive bilateral patchy infiltrates with small effusions are seen.

Fig. 5.**18    Haemophilus influenza pneumonia.** Poorly defined infiltrates are seen in both lower lobes (right posterior basal segment and left superior segment).

## Table 5.1    (Cont.) Alveolar Infiltrates and Atelectasis

| Disease | Radiographic Appearance | Comments |
|---|---|---|
| **Pneumonia, bacterial (cont.)** | | |
| **Bordetella pertussis** | Infiltrates conglomerate, often contiguous to the cardiac silhouette, producing a "shaggy heart sign." Mild hilar lymph node enlargement is occasionally associated. | Most common in nonimmunized children, but can occur in immunized adults. |
| **Francisella (Pasteurella) tularensis** | Unilateral or bilateral patchy to homogeneous consolidations, sometimes oval in shape. Ipsilateral hilar enlargement and pleural effusion are commonly associated. | Organism usually found in rodents and other small mammals. Tularemia often caused by occupational exposure (hunter, laboratory worker, butcher). |
| **Yersinia (Pasteurella) pestis** | Unilateral or bilateral homogeneous consolidations with air bronchograms. Hilar and paratracheal lymph node enlargement may be the dominant radiographic feature. Pleural effusions occur. | Organism still widespread among wild rodents. *Bacillus anthracis* (cattle, sheep and goats) may cause similar radiographic chest findings. Both anthrax and plague pneumonia are nowadays extremely rare diseases. |
| **Other Gram-negative aerobic bacteria (Fig. 5.19)** | Noncharacteristic, often nonhomogeneous infiltrate(s) in lower lobes. Cavitation occurs with varying frequency with most organisms. Pleural effusion may be present. | Organisms: *Bacillus proteus, Escherichia coli, Salmonella, Brucella, Enterobacter, Serratia,* and others. |
| **Bacteroides and other anaerobic bacteria** | Homogeneous infiltrate(s) preferentially in posterior segments with abscess formation early in the course characteristic, Pleural effusion (empyema) is very common. | Anaerobes are common organisms of normal flora of mouth and respiratory tract. Often found in "aspiration pneumonias" in alcoholics and people with poor oral hygiene. Course protracted over weeks to months. |
| **Tuberculosis (Mycobacterium tuberculosis) (Figs. 5.20 and 5.21)** | *Primary:* Consolidation with only slight predilection for upper lobes. Hilar and/or paratracheal lymph node enlargement is usually present. Pleural effusion is common in adults.<br>*Postprimary:* Patchy, inhomogeneous infiltrate in apical or posterior segments of upper lobes or superior segment of lower lobes is characteristic. Bilateral involvement is common, but often asymmetric. Pleural effusion and lymph node enlargement are rare. Cavitation occurs and may result in bronchogenic spread characterized by multiple patchy infiltrates. | Primary tuberculosis is often found in children.<br><br>In adults. Reactivation of an old focus, after BCG vaccination, or exogenous reinfection (rare), or as direct continuation of the original (primary) infection. |

*(continues on page 106)*

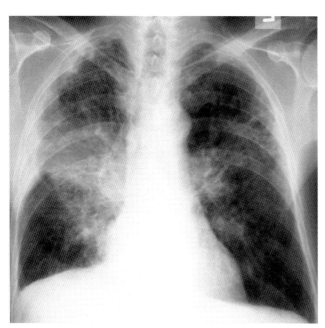

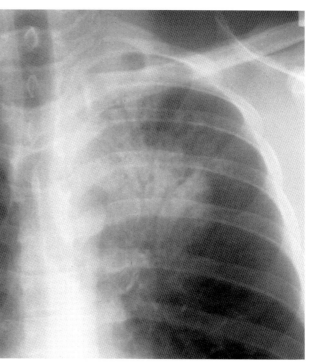

Fig. 5.**19    Serratia marcescens pneumonia.** Bilateral infiltrates with numerous small cavities and a larger consolidation in the right mid lung are seen. Small bilateral effusions, partially loculated along the right lateral chest wall, are also present.

Fig. 5.**20    Primary tuberculosis in AIDS.** A left upper lobe consolidation with air bronchogram and left hilar adenopathy is seen.

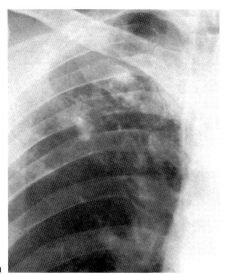

a

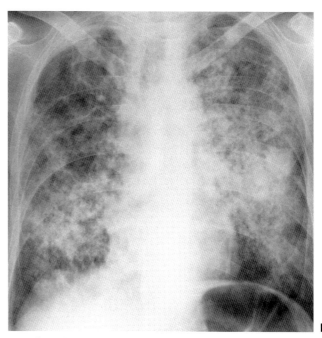

b

Fig. 5.**21 a, b    Postprimary tuberculosis** (2 cases). **a** A nonhomogeneous infiltrate is seen in the apical and posterior segment of the right upper lobe. **b** Cavitary tuberculosis with bronchogenic spread producing extensive confluent infiltrates bilaterally is evident.

## Table 5.1 (Cont.) Alveolar Infiltrates and Atelectasis

| Disease | Radiographic Appearance | Comments |
|---|---|---|
| *Pneumonia, bacterial* (cont.) | | |
| **Atypical mycobacteria (mycobacterium avium intracellulare or kansasii)** (Figs. 5.22 and 5.23 | Similar to tuberculosis, but greater tendency for cavitation, while pleural effusions and hilar adenopathy are less common. Strong association with preexisting pulmonary disease (e.g., emphysema, chronic bronchitis) and relatively common in AIDS. | Atypical mycobacteria can be isolated from the sputum of healthy people. Tuberculin test is negative and there is no response to antituberculous therapy. |
| **Actinomycosis Nocardiosis** (Figs. 5.24 and 5.25) | Homogeneous consolidation with lower lobe predilection. Cavitation and pleural effusion (empyema) are common. Extension through pleura into chest wall is frequent and often associated with rib destruction. | Whereas actinomycosis affects otherwise healthy people, nocardiosis is virtually limited to compromised hosts (e.g., diseases of reticuloendothelial system, immunosuppressive therapy, and alveolar proteinosis). |
| *Pneumonia, fungal* **Histoplasmosis** | *Primary:* Nonhomogeneous consolidations, most often in a lower lobe with hilar lymph enlargement are characteristic. A pleural effusion is rarely associated. *Postprimary:* Consolidations that clear in one area and appear in another are characteristic. Preferentially located in the upper lobes. Cavitation may occur. Lymph node enlargement is uncommon. | Clinical and radiographic features often resemble tuberculosis. |
| **Coccidioidomycosis** | Patchy homogeneous consolidations preferentially in lower lobes and often associated with hilar and/ or mediastinal lymph node enlargement and less commonly with a pleural effusion. Cavitation (usually thin-walled) occurs predominantly in the upper lobes, and unlike tuberculosis, involves also the anterior segments. | The disease is asymptomatic in the majority of infected patients or causes mild influenza-like symptoms. Endemic in southwest desert of USA, northern Mexico and in parts of Central and South America. |
| **Blastomycosis** | Nonspecific homogeneous or patchy consolidation, rarely associated with lymph node enlargement, pleural effusion and cavitation. | Caused by *Blastomyces dermatitidis* and found in North, Central, and South America and Africa. Also referred to as North American blastomycosis. |
| **Cryptococcosis** (Fig. 5.26) | Well-defined segmental or lobar consolidation preferentially in lower lobes. Cavitation and lymph node enlargement are rare. | Peripheral mass lesion is a more common radiographic presentation of this disease. Also referred to as torulosis or European blastomycosis. |
| **Mucormycosis (phycomycosis)** | Homogeneous consolidation, frequently with cavitation. | In patients with diabetes, lymphoma, or leukemia. |
| **Geotrichosis** | Consolidation in upper lobes, frequently associated with thin-walled cavities. | |
| **Sporotrichosis** | Segmental consolidations, commonly associated with hilar lymph node enlargement. Thin-walled cavities are not unusual. Spreading of the disease through pleura into the chest wall may occur. | The disease may also present radiographically as single large mass or as numerous small nodules. |
| **Aspergillosis** (Fig. 5.27) | Single or multiple consolidations. Abscess formation can occur. | Exceedingly rare in healthy patients (primary aspergillosis) but not unusual in compromised hosts ("aspergillosis with chronic debilitating disease"). Other manifestations of the disease include aspergillomas within pulmonary cavities and hypersensitivity aspergillosis (mucoid impaction especially in asthmatics, often simulating bronchogenic carcinoma radiographically). |
| **Candidiasis (moniliasis)** | Patchy infiltrates. Cavitation may occur. | Candida is a common saprophyte of upper respiratory tract. Common in elderly or persons with chronic debilitating disease. |

*(continues on page 108)*

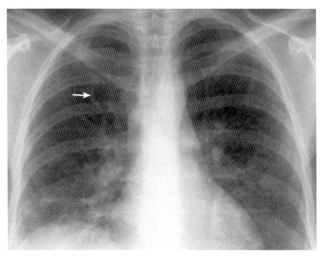

Fig. 5.**22**  **Atypical mycobacterial pneumonia.** Bilateral poorly defined nodular opacities predominantly involving the mid and lower lung zones are seen. A pneumatocele (arrow) is also evident in the right upper lobe.

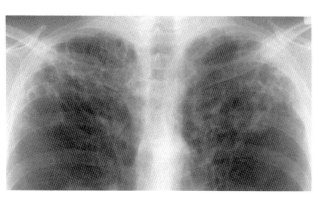

Fig. 5.**23**  **Atypical mycobacterial pneumonia.** Bilateral upper lobe infiltrates with numerous small thin-walled cavities are evident.

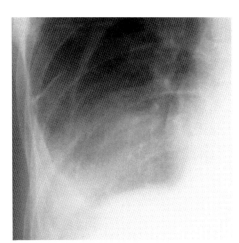

Fig. 5.**24**  **Pulmonary actinomycosis.** A right lower lobe consolidation with pleural reaction and extension into the adjacent ribs is seen.

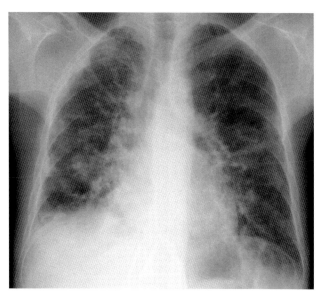

Fig. 5.**25**  **Pulmonary nocardiosis.** Multiple bilateral poorly defined nodular opacities often with cavitation are seen. A partially loculated right pleural effusion is also present.

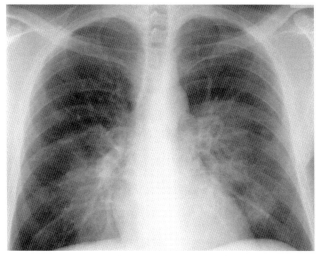

Fig. 5.**26**  **Cryptococcal pneumonia.** Bilateral, well defined homogeneous consolidations are seen in the lower lobes.

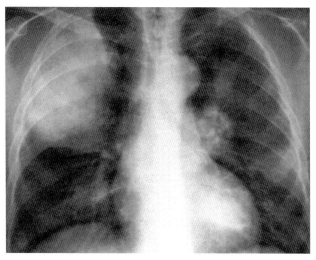

Fig. 5.**27**  **Pulmonary aspergillosis** in a patient with dermatomyositis treated with steroids, presenting with bilateral, rapidly increasing consolidations.

### Table 5.1    (Cont.) Alveolar Infiltrates and Atelectasis

| Disease | Radiographic Appearance | Comments |
|---|---|---|
| *Pneumonia, myco-plasma and viral*<br>    Mycoplasma<br>    Influenza<br>    Parainflueuza<br>    Coxsackie<br>    Adenovirus<br>    Psittacosis<br>    (Figs. 5.28, 5.29 and 5.30) | Patchy infiltrates, often preceded by fine reticular pattern and commonly located in one or both lower lobes, are characteristic. Small pleural effusions may be present. Cavitation does not occur and hilar lymph node enlargement is extremely rare in adults. | Common in children and young adults.<br>*Rubeola (measles)* and *echovirus pneumonias*, almost exclusively found in infants and young children, are commonly associated with hilar lymph node enlargement.<br>*Respiratory syncytial* virus infections are particularly common in infants and small children presenting with severe respiratory symptoms and only minimal radiographic findings (e.g., overinflation). |
| Mononucleosis (Epstein-Barr virus) | Similar to mycoplasma and aforementioned viral pneumonias, but hilar lymph node enlargement occurs. | Common disease in the 15–25-year age group, but pulmonary manifestations are rare. Usually associated with generalized lymphadenopathy and splenomegaly, the latter being often the most conspicuous radiographic feature. |
| Varicella (zoster) (Fig. 5.31 | Bilateral fluffy nodular infiltrates that may coalesce near the hilum when extensive and produce a "pulmonary edema"-type infiltrate. Lymph node enlargement and pleural effusions are rarely present. | Clinical symptoms and radiographic findings of chickenpox pneumonia occur 2–3 days after skin manifestation. |
| Cytomegalic inclusion disease (cytomegalovirus) (Fig. 5.32) | Patchy, often bilateral interstitial and alveolar infiltrates in advanced stage. Pleural effusion and cavitation do not occur. | In compromised hosts. Cytomegalovirus often coexistent with Pneumocystis carinii pneumonia. |
| SARS (Severe Acute Respiratory Distress Syndrome) (Fig. 5.33) | Unilateral or, slightly less common, bilateral, often multifocal airspace disease with lower lobe predilection. Pleural effusions are uncommon at initial presentation. | Highly contagious viral pneumonia with 10 % mortality rate. |
| *Pneumonia, rickettsial*<br>    Q-fever (Coxiella burnetii) | Homogeneous consolidation involving an entire segment (usually in a lower lobe) is characteristic. Pleural reaction may be present. | Disease clinically simulates influenza. Chest radiographs abnormal in less than 50 % of patients. |

*(continues on page 110)*

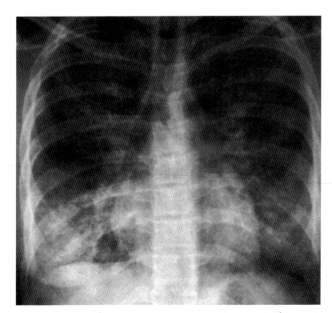

Fig. 5.**28**   **Mycoplasma pneumonia** presenting as mixed interstitial and alveolar infiltrates in the right middle lobe and both lower lobes.

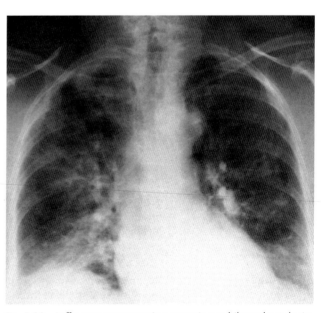

Fig. 5.**29**   **Influenza pneumonia** presenting as bilateral patchy infiltrates.

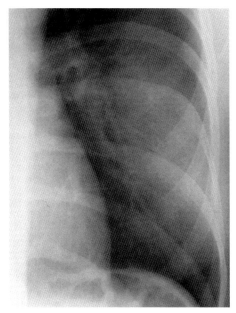

Fig. 5.**30**  **Psittacosis pneumonia.** A homogeneous "ground-glass" opacity in the left lower lobe is associated with mild left hilar adenopathy. This is a relatively unique presentation of the disease that often presents in a less characteristic, viral pneumonia pattern.

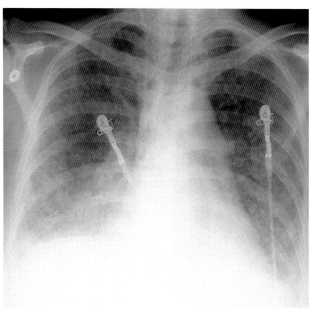

Fig. 5.**31**  **Varicella pneumonia.** Bilateral fluffy nodular infiltrates that coalesce in the lower lobes are seen.

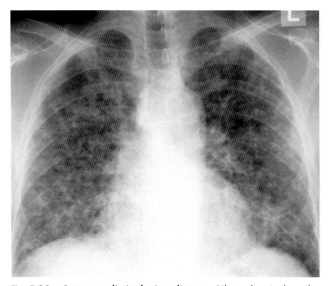

Fig. 5.**32**  **Cytomegalic inclusion disease.** Bilateral reticulonodular and early alveolar infiltrates are seen mainly involving the mid and lower lung zones.

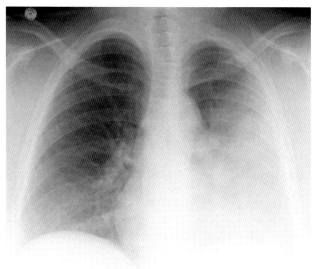

Fig. 5.**33**  **SARS.** A poorly defined consolidation involving the lingula and left lower lobe is seen.

### Table 5.1 (Cont.) Alveolar Infiltrates and Atelectasis

| Disease | Radiographic Appearance | Comments |
| --- | --- | --- |
| **Asbestosis (Fig. 5.38)** | Combination of parenchymal and pleural changes in mid and lower-lung fields results in partial obliteration of the heart border ("shaggy heart" sign) and diaphragm. Parietal pleural plaques, which may be calcified, may be present and are characteristic. | High incidence of associated malignancies such as mesothelioma, bronchogenic and alveolar cell carcinomas. |
| **Talcosis** | Pulmonary (reticulonodular pattern with homogeneous, poorly defined infiltrates) and pleural changes (plaques) similar to asbestosis. | |
| **Aspiration of solid foreign body** | Localized , gravity-dependent consolidation and atelectasis, most often in lower lobes. Abscess formation is common. | If the foreign body produces a check-valve mechanism, hyperinflation and air trapping can be seen distally to it. The foreign body occasionally can be identified when radiopaque or outlined by air. |
| **Aspiration, acute** | Confluent patchy infiltrates to homogeneous consolidations, often bilateral. | Aspiration of gastric contents (*Mendelson's syndrome*) usually results in bilateral infiltrates that clear in 7 to 10 days. |
| **Aspiration, chronic** | One or more segmental consolidation (s) slowly clearing in one area and appearing in consolidation(s) another. | Encountered with Zenker's diverticulum, esophageal stenosis, tracheoesophageal fistula and neuromuscular disorders.<br>Acute and chronic aspiration pneumonias are also found in alcoholics. |
| **Lipoid pneumonia (exogenous)** | Relatively homogeneous consolidations in one or more segments preferentially in lower lobes. Interstitial thickening, evident as linear densities in the periphery of the lesion, may be found. | Aspiration of oil (e.g., oily nose drops). *Endogenous lipoid pneumonias* (e.g., cholesterol pneumonia, and primary or secondary inflammatory pseudotumors, the latter in association with pre-existing lung disease) must be differentiated. |
| **Lymphocytic interstitial pneumonia (Fig. 5.39)** | Bilateral reticulonodular or, less commonly, ground glass opacities and consolidations with preferential involvement of the lower lung zones. Hilar and mediastinal lymphadenopathy may be associated in patients with AIDS. | Patients usually have underlying diseases such as rheumatoid arthritis, Sjögren's syndrome or AIDS, in which children typically are affected. |
| **Mucoid impaction (hypersensitivity aspergillosis) (Fig. 5.40)** | Mucous plugs often recognizable as "broad band"-like, V- or Y-shaped densities preferentially in upper lobes. Atelectasis or obstructive pneumonitis often present distally to the plug, simulating a neoplasm. May clear in one area and reappear in another. | Usually associated with asthma and/or chronic bronchial disease (e.g., bronchiectasis, cystic fibrosis). Peripheral eosinophilia commonly found in mucoid impaction caused by hypersensitivity (allergic) aspergillosis.<br>*Bronchocentric granulomatosis (Liebow)* presents clinically and radiographically similar to mucoid impaction and may be considered a variant of that entity. |

*(continues on page 114)*

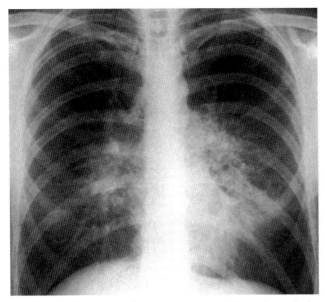

Fig. 5.**38 Pulmonary asbestosis** causing obliteration of the heart border ("shaggy heart" sign).

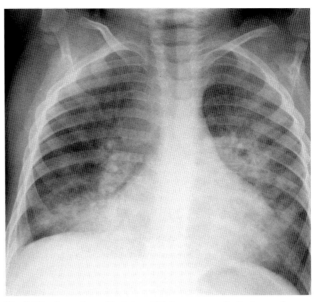

Fig. 5.**39 Lymphocytic interstitial pneumonia in transplacental AIDS.** Bilateral consolidations in the mid and lower lung zones are associated with hilar and right mediastinal adenopathy.

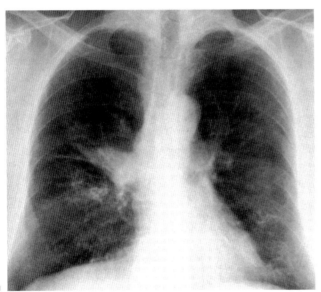

a

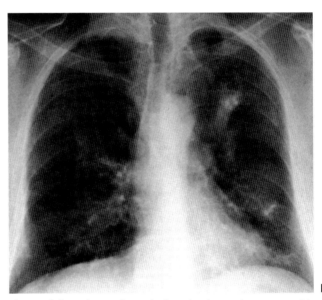

b

Fig. 5.**40 a, b Mucoid impaction (hypersensitivity aspergillosis)** in a patient with chronic lung disease. **a** Atelectasis and obstructive pneumonitis in the right middle lobe caused by a mucous plug are followed several months later by obstructive pneumonitis secondary to a plug in the left upper lobe seen in **b**.

## Table 5.1    (Cont.) Alveolar Infiltrates and Atelectasis

| Disease | Radiographic Appearance | Comments |
|---|---|---|
| **Loeffler's syndrome** (Fig. 5.41 and 5.42) | One or several poorly defined transient consolidations in the lung periphery are characteristic ("reversed pulmonary edema pattern"). | Blood eosinophilia is almost invariably present. May be idiopathic, drug-induced (e.g., penicillin, sulfonamides) or parasite-induced. A chronic form (*"chronic eosinophilic pneumonia"*) that is radiographically indistinguishable but persists for weeks when not treated with steroids, can be differentiated from the (acute) Loeffler's syndrome. |
| **Bronchiolitis obliterans organizing pneumonia (BOOP)** (Fig. 5.43) | Four distinctive patterns are discerned: 1. Multiple bilateral patchy consolidations. 2. Diffuse bilateral reticulonodular infiltrates. 3. Focal consolidation. 4. Multiple large nodules. | May be idiopathic (cryptogenic) or associated with connective tissue disease, drugs, infection and aspiration. Present clinically as a subacute illness with cough (90%), dyspnea (80%), fever (60%) and weight loss (50%). |
| **Connective tissue disease** (Fig. 5.44) | Nonspecific patchy peripheral consolidations often associated with pleural effusions. | In systemic lupus erythematosus and polyarteritis nodosa, for example. |
| **Wegener's granulomatosis** (Fig. 5.45) | Patchy infiltrates or a relatively homogeneous consolidation involving part of a segment to an entire lobe are well-recognized but not very common manifestations of this disease. Pleural reactions can occasionally be associated. | Most commonly found in middle-aged men, slightly less common in women. Pulmonary nodules which may cavitate are the characteristic radiographic presentation of this disease. |
| **Pulmonary infarct** (Fig. 5.46) | Pleural based consolidation(s), preferentially in lower lobes, which is often associated with pleural effusion and the elevation of ipsilateral diaphragm. *Hampton's hump* is characteristic but not common: The infarct appears as a truncated cone with its base contiguous to the visceral pleura. | Time of resolution varies between a few days (when only edema and/or hemorrhage is present) to several weeks (when associated with necrosis). Characteristically, a resolving infarct gradually diminishes but maintains the original shape and homogeneity ("melting ice cube" sign). |
| **Pulmonary edema (cardiogenic and non-cardiogenic)** | Nonsymmetrical, atypical presentation as areas of localized consolidations occurs in patients with pre-existing lung disease. | For differential diagnosis see Chapter 7. |

*(continues on page 116)*

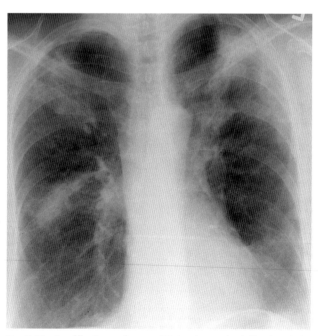

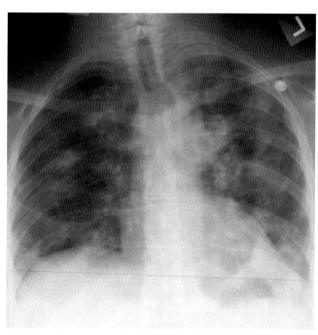

Fig. 5.**41    Loeffler's syndrome.** Bilateral, poorly defined, patchy infiltrates are seen in the periphery of the mid and upper lung zones in this patient with chronic obstructive pulmonary disease (COPD).

Fig. 5.**42    Chronic eosinophilic pneumonia.** Multiple, bilateral, poorly defined, patchy infiltrates are evident.

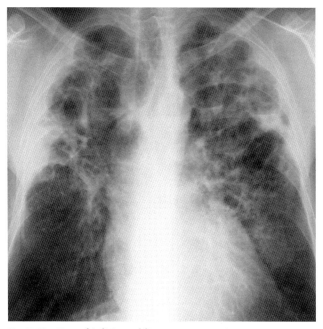

Fig. 5.**43 Bronchiolitis obliterans organizing pneumonia (BOOP).** Bilateral patchy infiltrates mainly involving the mid and upper lung zones are superimposed on chronic pulmonary changes including fibrosis ("honeycombing"), cystic bronchiectasis and bullous emphysema as well as chronic pleural disease.

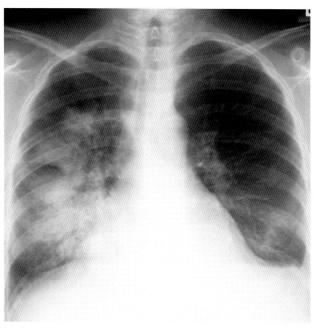

Fig. 5.**44 Lupus pneumonitis.** A large dense, poorly defined consolidation in the right perihilar and mid-lung zone is associated with an early left lower lower infiltrate and small left pleural reaction. Because of the patient's hemoptysis and absence of infection the underlying cause was considered to be extensive alveolar hemorrhage.

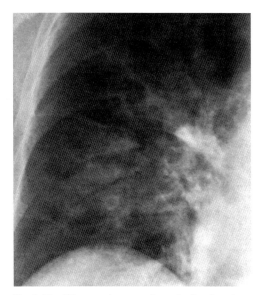

Fig. 5.**45 Wegener's granulomatosis.** An air-space consolidation involving mainly the right lower lobe is seen. Similar but less severe infiltrates were also present in the left tower lobe,

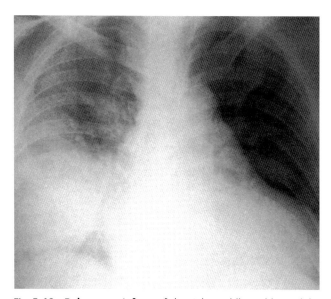

Fig. 5.**46 Pulmonary infarct** of the right middle and lower lobe in a patient with arteriosclerotic heart disease presenting as large consolidation.

## Table 5.1    (Cont.) Alveolar Infiltrates and Atelectasis

| Disease | Radiographic Appearance | Comments |
|---|---|---|
| **Pulmonary hemorrhage (nontraumatic)** (Fig. 5.47) | Usually bilateral alveolar densities clearing 2–3 days after single bleeding episode. | E.g. in *bleeding diathesis, idiopathic pulmonary hemosiderosis* and *Goodpasture's syndrome.* |
| **Pulmonary contusion** | Patchy infiltrates to extensive homogeneous consolidations apparent within 6 hours after trauma. Resolution begins rapidly and is completed within 3–7 days. | Usually in lung adjacent to the traumatized area but occasionally in the opposite lung (contre coup effect). |
| **Bronchial fracture** (Fig. 5.48) | Opacification (atelectasis) of a lobe or even an entire lung. May not become evident until months after traumatic episode, when bronchial stenosis develops at fracture side. Besides a pneumothorax, a localized to extensive pneumomediastinum is a common initial finding. Fractures of the first three ribs are very often associated in the adult. | Pneumothorax is usually the most striking finding but not present in 30% of cases, when fracture is incomplete or affects a bronchus within the mediastinum. |
| **Lung torsion** | Exudation of blood causes opacification ot the entire lung, that is rotated 180 degrees. Alteration in pulmonary vasculature characteristic. | Almost invariably in children. |
| **Radiation pneumonitis** (Fig. 5.49) | Consolidation often with air bronchograms developing 1 month to 1 year (most commonly 2–4 months) after cessation of radiation therapy. Localization corresponds to irradiated area. The fibrotic stage is usually present at 9–12 months and characterized by significant loss of volume, dense strands, and opacification of the involved area. Radiation-induced pleural effusions are unusual but pleural thickening is relatively common. | Radiation effect depends on total dose, number of fractions, and time elapsed between first and last treatment. A dose of at least 20 Gy is usually required, whereas doses of 60 Gy administered over 6 weeks almost always cause a severe radiation pneumonitis. |

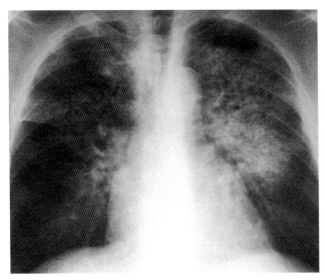

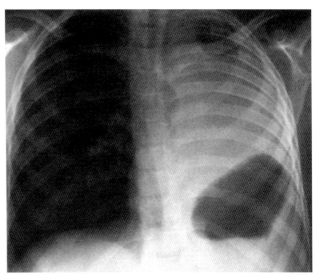

Fig. 5.**47   Pulmonary hemorrhage in idiopathic pulmonary hemosiderosis.** Bilateral alveolar densities with predominantly perihilar distribution are seen.

Fig. 5.**48   Bronchial fracture.** Atelectasis of the left lung is evident.

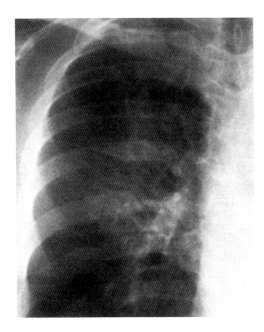

Fig. 5.**49   Radiation pneumonitis.** An infiltrate in the anteromedial portions of the right upper and mid lung field is seen, corresponding to the radiation ports for breast carcinoma.

# 6 Interstitial Lung Disease

Interstitial lung disease is diagnosed radiographically when a *reticular, nodular,* or *honeycomb pattern* or any combination thereof is recognizable.

The *reticular pattern* consists of a network of linear densities (Fig. 6.1 a). Depending on the mesh size, one can distinguish between fine, medium, and coarse reticular patterns, although this distinction has no obvious differential diagnostic significance. Kerley lines refer to septal lines that are thickened either by fluid accumulation, cellular infiltration, or connective tissue proliferation within the interlobular septa. Acute or transient Kerley lines are usually found with hydrostatic pulmonary edema (elevated microvascular pressure caused by left ventricular failure, renal disease and fluid overload), and occasionally with pneumonia and pulmonary hemorrhage. Acute Kerley lines are frequently associated with prominent interlobar fissures caused by subpleural edema. Permanent Kerley lines are most often present in chronic and severe pulmonary venous hypertension (especially mitral stenosis) that eventually results in fibrosis and hemosiderin deposition within the interlobular septa. Lymphatic obstruction appears to be a major factor in the development of Kerley lines associated with malignancies (e.g., lymphangitic carcinomatosis, bronchogenic carcinoma, and lymphoma), since at least histologically, ipsilateral hilar involvement with tumor is almost invariably present under such conditions. Finally, fibrosis of the interlobular septa can be associated with any form of pulmonary fibrosis, but is most frequently observed with pneumoconiosis.

Different kinds of Kerley lines are distinguished: Kerley A lines are straight lines measuring 2–6 cm in length and approximately 1 mm in thickness. They are located in radiating fashion midway between the hilum and pleura and appear to cross over bronchoarterial bundles showing no anatomic relationship with the latter. Kerley A lines are usually best seen in the mid and lower lung fields. Kerley B lines are thinner and shorter than Kerley A lines (up to 2 cm) and lie in the lung periphery perpendicular to the lateral pleural surface (Fig. 6.1 b). They are most numerous at the base of the lungs. *Plate-like (discoid) atelectases and localized fibrotic strands* can be differentiated from Kerley lines by their lack of a characteristic anatomic location and by the great variation in length and width of these densities.

A nodular pattern (Fig. 6.1 c) consists of numerous punctate densities essentially ranging in diameter from 1 mm (barely visible as an individual lesion) to 5 mm, although a few slightly larger nodular lesions can be interspersed. A purely nodular pattern is found with the hematogenous spread of certain infections and tumors, but can also be encountered with other diseases (Table 6.1). More often, however, nodular and reticular patterns are combined in the same patient, resulting in a *reticulonodular appearance* of the interstitial disease.

A *ground-glass appearance* (Fig. 6.1 d) is caused by a hazy increase in lung density that is not associated with obscuration of underlying vascular markings. It is found, besides in interstitial diseases, also with air-space disease (e.g. pneumocystis carinii pneumonia) and increased capillary blood volume (e.g. congestive heart failure). In interstitial disease it is produced when the fine reticulogranular pattern has progressed to such an extent that the overall density of the involved lung is increased, but the individual interstitial lesion is no longer recognizable.

A *honeycomb pattern* is characterized by round or oval cystic lesions with a diameter up to 1 cm (Fig. 6.1e). In a given patient, they are relatively uniform in size and usually bunched together in grape-like clusters. Honeycombing is the only dependable radiographic sign of *interstitial fibrosis.* It may present radiographically in a reticulonodular pattern, too, but this presentation is also found with many other disorders, including various acute abnormalities that can resolve completely with time. *Cystic bronchiectases* may produce a radiographic picture similar to honeycombing. However, they can usually be differentiated from honeycombing by their larger and less uniform size and by the presence of tiny meniscus-like fluid levels at the bottom of these cystic lesions. Diseases that cause a characteristic honeycomb pattern are summarized in Table 6.2.

The majority of interstitial lung diseases involve both lungs, or stated differently, the interstitial disease is usually diffuse, although some areas may be more affected and others more or less spared. Truly *localized interstitial lung disease* is relatively rare and most often of an infectious etiology. *Mycoplasma* and *viral pneumonias* can present in their early stages as localized interstitial diseases of fine reticular appearance before the extension of the inflammation into the air spaces causes a consolidation. Localized fibrotic changes are often found in the chronic stage of a disease (e. g., *tuberculosis* and *radiation pneumonitis*). Finally, fibrotic scars may be the sequelae of virtually any disease capable of damaging the lung parenchyma severely enough.

Both congenital and acquired *bronchiectases* can be mistaken radiographically for localized interstitial lung disease (Fig. 6.1f). In approximately 50 % of cases, they are limited to one lung. Cylindrical bronchiectases present as tubular opacities with parallel walls of 1 mm or slightly larger thickness. When these bronchiectatic segments become filled with retained secretion, they appear as homogeneous band-like densities ("gloved-finger" shadows). Varicose and cystic (saccular) bronchiectases are often evident on plain radiography as cystic lesions up to 2 cm in diameter and often containing a small air-fluid level at the bottom. This appearance is virtually diagnostic, although under very rare circumstances both pulmonary papillomatosis and paragonimiasis may mimic cystic bronchiectases. Bronchiectases are often associated with loss of volume and crowding of the lung markings in the affected area together with compensatory overinflation of the spared lung (Fig. 6.2).

Table 6.3 summarizes all disorders that demonstrate radiographically a diffuse reticular or reticulonodular pattern characteristic of interstitial lung disease.

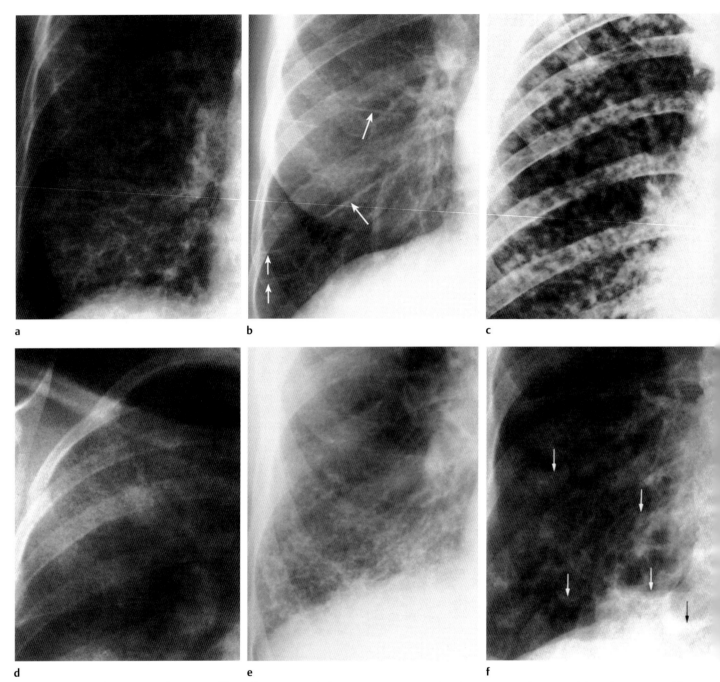

a  b  c

d  e  f

Fig. 6.**1 a–f** **Patterns of interstitial lung disease. a** Reticular pattern (Pneumocystis carinii pneumonia). **b** Kerley A lines (long arrows, touched up) and Kerley B lines (short arrows) (mitral stenosis). **c** Nodular pattern (silicosis). **d** Ground-glass appearance produced by the summation of innumerable tiny retlculogranular densities (sarcoidosis). **e** Honeycomb pattern (idiopathic interstitial fibrosis). **f** Bronchiectases evident as cystic lesions varying considerably in size and characteristically containing small air-fluid levels (arrows).

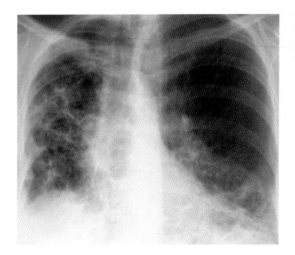

Fig. 6.**2** **Bronchiectases.** Extensive, predominantly cystic bronchiectases in the right lung and left lower lobe are associated with loss of volume in the affected lung and compensatory overinflation of the nonaffected left upper lobe.

**Table 6.1 Disseminated Pulmonary Nodules Measuring Less than 1 cm in Diameter ("Miliary" is defined as 1–3 mm in diameter)**

| Disease | Characteristics of Nodules |
|---|---|
| **Bronchioloalveolar carcinoma (alveolar cell carcinoma) (Fig 6.3)** | Often poorly defined, confluent nodules of varying size. Roentgenographic pattern of disseminated alveolar cell carcinoma may be fairly uniform throughout both lungs or vary regionally. |
| **Metastases (e.g., carcinomas from thyroid, lung, breast or gastrointestinal tract, or melanomas, sarcomas and lymphomas) (Fig. 6.4)** | Usually well defined and of varying size. |
| *Pneumonias* | |
| Staphylococcus aureus | Miliary and larger, often poorly defined; can form microabscesses. |
| Salmonella | Miliary. |
| Pseodomonas pseudomallei | 4 to 10 mm, poorly defined (early acute stage of disease). |
| Listeriosis (newborn) | Intrauterine infection with high mortality rate. |

*(continues on page 122)*

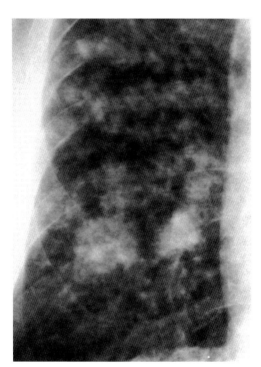

Fig. 6.**3 Bronchioloalveolar carcinoma.** Poorly defined, confluent nodules are seen bilaterally, but only shown for the right side.

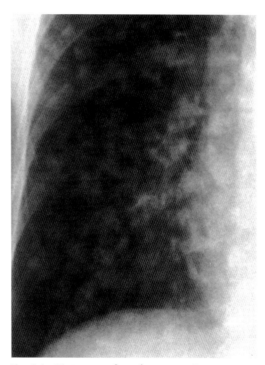

Fig. 6.**4 Metastases from breast carcinoma.** Numerous nodules measuring only a few millimeters in diameter are present bilaterally, but are only shown for the right lower lung field.

**Table 6.1   (Cont.) Disseminated Pulmonary Nodules Measuring Less than 1 cm in Diameter ("Miliary" is defined as 1–3 mm in diameter)**

| Disease | Characteristics of Nodules |
| --- | --- |
| **Tuberculosis** (Fig. 6.5) | Miliary, discrete (DD: tuberculomas that are larger than 5 mm and can calcify). |
| **Histoplasmosis** (Fig 6.6) | 2 to 4 mm, discrete. Can result in nodular calcifications 1 to several years later. |
| **Coccidioidomycosis, blastomycosis, and Cryptococcosis (Fig. 6.7)** | Miliary and larger (up to 3 cm). Calcification extremely rare. |
| **Candidiasis** | Miliary (rare manifestation) |
| **Varicella (chickenpox) pneumonia** (Fig. 6.8) | Miliary and larger, poorly defined. Healing may result in punctate calcifications years later, |
| **Schistosomiasis** | Miliary |
| **Filariasis** | Miliary and slightly larger (up to 5 mm). Predominantly in the mid- and lower-lung fields. |

*(continues on page 124)*

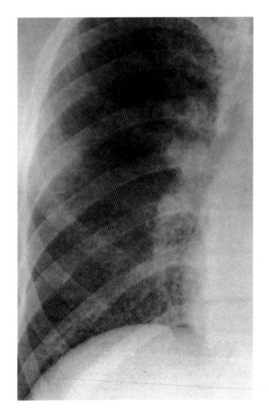

Fig. 6.**5**   **Miliary tuberculosis.** Numerous discrete nodules measuring 1 to 3 mm in diameter are seen bilaterally, but are only shown for the right side.

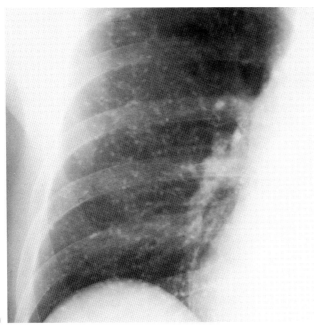
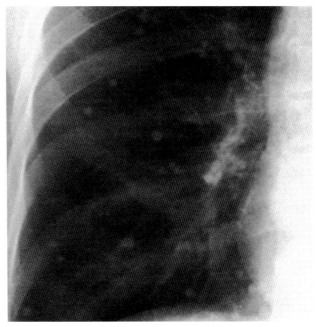

a

b

Fig. 6.**6** **Histoplasmosis (2 cases).** Bilateral miliary (**a**) and larger (**b**) scattered calcified nodules are present, but only shown for the right side.

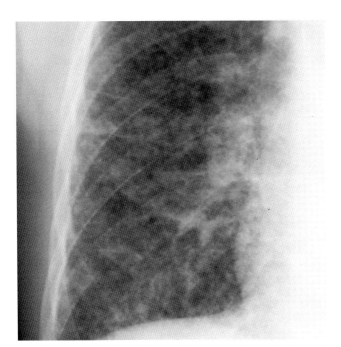

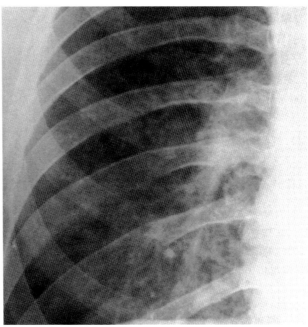

Fig. 6.**7** **Aspergillosis.** Diffuse bilateral poorly defined small nodular densities are present, but only shown for the right lower lung field.

Fig. 6.**8** **Varicella (chickenpox) pneumonia.** Poorly defined nodular densities are seen bilaterally, but are only shown for the right lower lung field.

**Table 6.1   (Cont.) Disseminated Pulmonary Nodules Measuring Less than 1 cm in Diameter ("Miliary" is defined as 1–3 mm in diameter)**

| Disease | Characteristics of Nodules |
|---|---|
| Sarcoidosis (Fig. 6.9) | Miliary and larger, often indistinctly defined. |
| Pneumoconiosis (inorganic dust) (e.g., silicosis, coal miner's lung, berylliosis) (Figs. 6.10 and 6.11) | Miliary and larger. Fairly well defined in silicosis and poorly in berylliosis. Calcification occurs. |
| Pneumoconiosis caused by radiopaque dusts (iron, tin, barium, antimony and rare-earth compounds) (Figs. 6.12 and 6.13) | Finely granular stippling uniformly distributed over both lung fields. Density of the tiny nodules depends on the atomic number of the inhaled element. |
| Silo filler's disease ($NO_2$ inhalation) | Miliary nodulation only manifest 2–5 weeks after initial exposure (third phase of disease). |
| Extrinsic allergic alveolitis (e.g., farmer's lung, bird-fancier's lung, mushroom-worker's lung, bagassosis, and others) (Figs. 6.14 and 6.15) | Miliary and larger, usually poorly defined (acute stage). Often less evident in apices and bases. |
| Rheumatoid lung | Miliary and larger (in early stage). |
| Wegener's granulomatosis | Multiple nodules ranging from a few millimeters up to 10 cm. |

*(continues on page 126)*

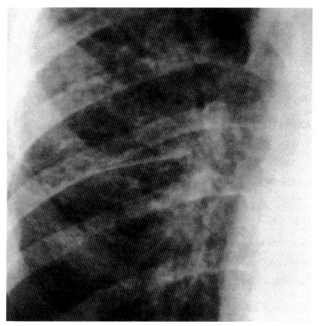

Fig. 6.**9   Sarcoidosis.** Multiple small nodules of variable sizes are seen bilaterally, but are only shown for the right mid lung field.

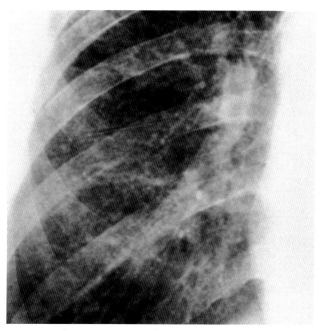

Fig. 6.**10   Silicosis.** Numerous fairly well defined miliary nodules are seen bilaterally besides diffuse reticular changes and early honeycombing, but are only shown for the right side.

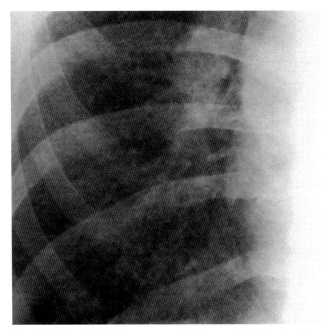

Fig. 6.**11** **Berylliosis.** Numerous relatively poorly defined miliary nodules and bilateral hilar enlargement are present, but are only shown for the right side. Findings simulate sarcoidosis radiographically.

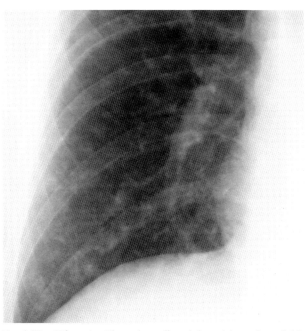

Fig. 6.**12** **Siderosis.** Bilateral small nodules with preferential involvement of the mid and lower lung zones are seen in this arc welder that are not associated with hilar adenopathy or fibrosis and resolved after exposure was discontinued. Only the right lower lung field is shown.

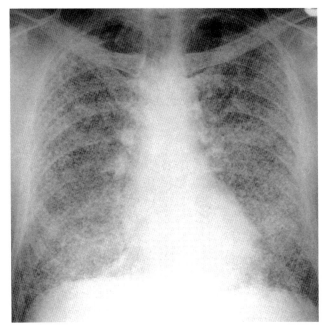

Fig. 6.**13** **Stannosis** (inhalation of tin oxide). Multiple tiny nodules of high density are distributed evenly throughout both lungs, sparing only the apices.

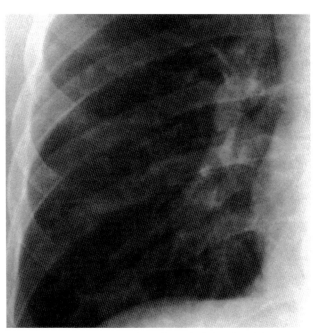

Fig. 6.**14** **Farmer's lung.** Bilateral poorly defined nodules are present.

**Table 6.1 (Cont.) Disseminated Pulmonary Nodules Measuring Less than 1 cm in Diameter ("Miliary" is defined as 1–3 mm in diameter)**

| Disease | Characteristics of Nodules |
|---|---|
| Langerhans cell histiocytosis (eosinophilic granuloma) (Fig. 6.16) | Miliary and larger with mid and upper lung fields predominance. This presentation is seen in the active stage, which may completely resolve or progress to the chronic fibrotic stage. |
| Gaucher's disease | Miliary and larger. |
| Niemann-Pick syndrome | Miliary and larger. |
| Interstitial edema (cardiogenic) | Symmetrical, miliary nodulation, preferentially located in the lower-lung fields. May occasionally be the dominant feature. |
| Hemosiderosis and pulmonary ossification secondary to mitral stenosis (Fig. 6.17) | Punctate densities (hemosiderosis) and densely calcified 2 to 8 mm nodules (pulmonary ossification), predominantly in the mid and lower lung fields, usually more numerous on the right side. Hemosiderosis-like pulmonary calcifications are occasionally seen in chronic renal failure (see Fig. 7.29). |
| Bronchiolitis acute or obliterans | Miliary and larger |
| Amyloidosis (diffuse alveolar septal form) | Miliary and larger |
| Talc granulomatosis secondary to intravenous drug abuse | Discrete, 1 mm and smaller, may slowly increase in size and number over months and years. |
| Alveolar microlithiasis (Fig. 6.18) | Discrete and extremely sharply defined, less than 1 mm in diameter. |
| Oily contrast material embolism (e.g., secondary to lymphography) (Fig. 6.19) | Finely granular and relatively dense stippling preferentially located in the posterior (dependent) parts of the lungs and most obvious a few hours after lymphography. |

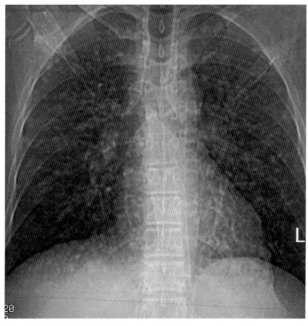

Fig. 6.**15 Bird-fancier's lung.** Multiple small nodules are scattered throughout both lung fields.

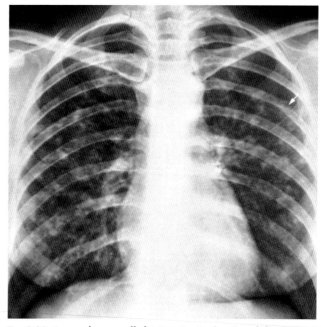

Fig. 6.**16 Langerhans cell histiocytosis (eosinophilic granuloma).** Multiple poorly defined nodules are seen bilaterally. Note also the lytic involvement of the left fifth rib with pathologic fracture (arrow).

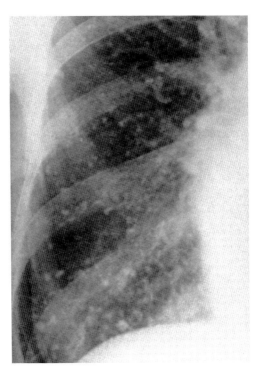
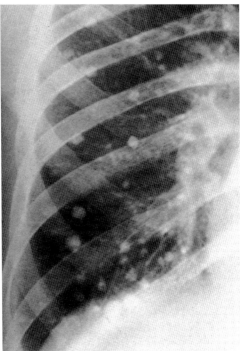

Fig. 6.**17**  **Mitral stenosis** (2 cases). **a** Punctate densities (hemosiderosis), and **b** larger calcified nodules (pulmonary ossification) are seen bilaterally, but only shown for the right side.

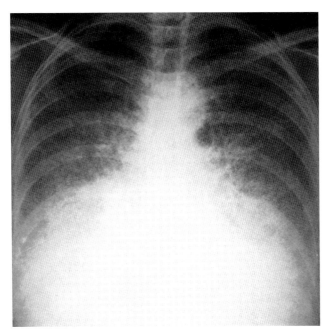
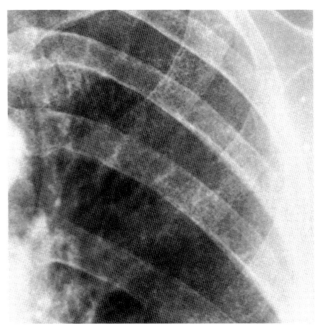

Fig. 6.**18**  **Alveolar microlithiasis.** Innumerable, extremely sharply defined, tiny densities measuring less than 1 mm in diameter are seen bilaterally.

Fig. 6.**19**  **Oily contrast material embolism after lymphography.** Finely granular and relatively dense stippling is seen throughout both lungs, but only shown for the left upper lung field.

## Table 6.2 Honeycombing

| Disease | Comments |
| --- | --- |
| **Pneumoconiosis** (silicosis, coal miner's lung, asbestosis, berylliosis, and others.) (Fig. 6.20) | Usually associated with other manifestations (nodules; conglomerate masses, hilar enlargement, etc). Lung volume normal or increased (emphysema). |
| Sarcoidosis (Fig. 6.21) | Persisting hilar and mediastinal lymphadenopathy often present. Lung volume normal or increased (emphysema). |
| Tuberculosis (Fig. 6.22) | A localized honeycombing pattern in the upper lobes can be simulated by tuberculous bronchiectasis and fibrosis. |
| **Langerhans cell histiocytosis (eosinophilic granuloma)** (Fig. 6.23) | Honeycombing characteristically more prominent in upper and mid lung fields and sparing the lung bases. Lung volume normal. Spontaneous pneumothorax occurs relatively frequently. |

*(continues on page 129)*

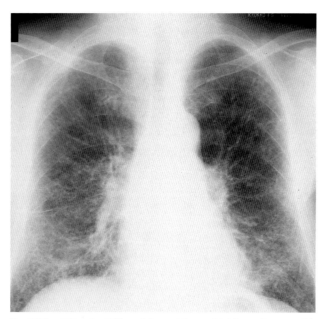

Fig. 6.**20** **Silicosis.** Diffuse bilateral interstitial lung disease with extensive fibrosis (honeycombing) is present.

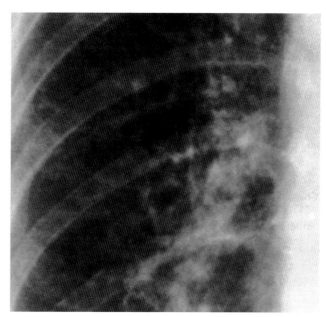

Fig. 6.**21** **Sarcoidosis.** Reticulonodular disease with early honeycombing is seen bilaterally, but only shown for the right mid lung field.

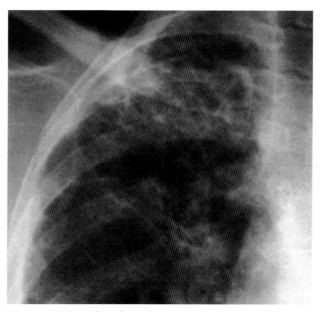

Fig. 6.**22** **Tuberculous bronchiectasis.** A honeycomb pattern is simulated by the bronchiectatic changes in both upper lobes, but more pronounced on the right side shown here.

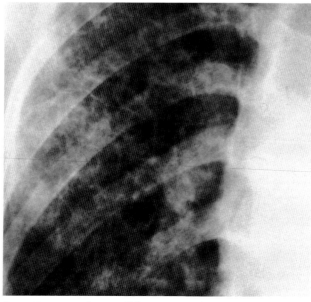

Fig. 6.**23** **Langerhans cell histiocytosis (eosinophilic granuloma).** Pulmonary fibrosis evident as honeycombing is predominantly involving the mid and upper lung fields.

## Table 6.2 (Cont.) Honeycombing

| Disease | Comments |
|---|---|
| Connective tissue disease (especially scleroderma and rheumatoid lung) (Figs. 6.24 and 6.25) | Honeycombing usually most prominent at the bases. Progressive loss of lung volume is characteristically associated, particularly in scleroderma. |
| Idiopathic pulmonary fibrosis ("usual" interstitial pneumonia [UIP], Hamman-Rich syndrome) (Fig. 6.26) | Honeycombing usually most prominent at the bases. Progressive loss of lung volume characteristic. (Radiographically indistinguishable from scleroderma). |
| | Diffuse interstitial fibrosis, similar to the idiopathic form, may represent the end stage of a variety of pulmonary conditions (e.g., *drug induced*, especially by busulfan, bleomycin, methotrexate), *inhalation of noxious gases* and *organic dusts* (e.g., farmer's lung), *chronic or recurrent pulmonary edema,*especially in mitral valve disease, and others. Radiographically, however, an unequivocal honeycombing pattern is rarely found in these conditions. |

(continues on page 130)

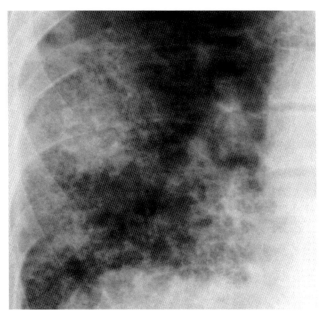

Fig. 6.**24** **Scleroderma.** Honeycombing and loss of lung volume, evident by the high diaphragms bilaterally, are present, but only shown for the right lower lung field.

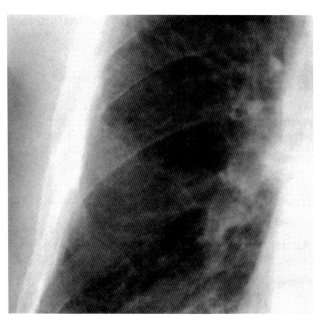

Fig. 6.**25** **Rheumatoid lung disease.** Reticulonodular disease with honeycombing is present, but only shown for the right lower lung field.

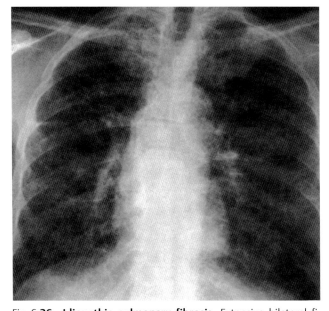

Fig. 6.**26** **Idiopathic pulmonary fibrosis.** Extensive bilateral fibrosis with honeycombing and loss of lung volume is seen.

### Table 6.2 (Cont.) Honeycombing

| Disease | Comments |
|---|---|
| Desquamative interstitial pneumonitis (DIP) (Fig. 6.27) | Honeycombing indistinguishable from idiopathic pulmonary fibrosis (base predominance and loss of volume) is found in end-stage DIP. Ground-glass opacification and loss of definitions of basal vascular markings are often associated and quite characteristic. |
| Lipoid pneumonia (exogenous) | Rare. Localized honeycombing usually located in a lower lobe. |
| Amyloidosis | Rare. Honeycombing preferentially in lower lobes. Hilar and mediastinal adenopathy may be associated. |
| Ankylosing spondylitis with upper lobe pulmonary fibrosis | Rare. Exclusively located in upper lobes. Resembles upper lobe fibrosis and bronchiectasis secondary to tuberculosis. |
| Tuberous sclerosis | Rare. Predominantly lower lobe involvement. Diffuse honeycombing represents the end stage of pulmonary manifestations. Lung volume is normal or increased (associated emphysema). Chylous pleural effusions are often associated. Sclerotic bone lesions may be evident. |
| Lymphangiomyomatosis (lymphangioleiomyomatosis) (Fig. 6.28) | Rare, nonfamilial disease exclusively found in females of childbearing age, with pulmonary and pleural manifestations indistinguishable from tuberous sclerosis. |
| Neurofibromatosis | Rare. Pulmonary fibrosis and bullae are often combined. Skin nodules, scoliosis, rib notching and mediastinal masses may also be evident. |
| Gaucher's disease | Rare. Splenomegaly and bony changes (e.g. osteopenia, compression fractures in the thoracic spine and osteonecrosis in long bones) may be associated. |
| NiemannPick disease | Rare. Splenomegaly and bony changes in the thoracic spine similar to Gaucher's disease. |

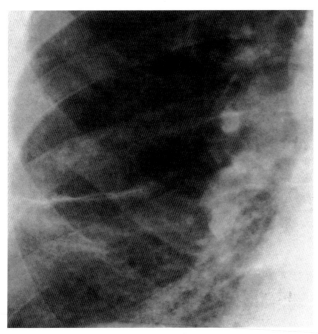

Fig. 6.**27** **Desquamative interstitial pneumonitis.** Interstitial disease producing ground-glass appearance and honeycombing is particularly pronounced in the lower lung fields, but only shown for the right side. A loss of definition of the basal vascular markings is also evident.

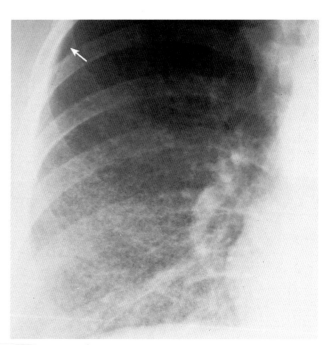

Fig. 6.**28** **Lymphangiomyomatosis.** Diffuse bilateral interstitial disease with a fine honeycomb pattern is evident in the mid and lower lung zones, but only shown for the right side. A small pneumothorax (arrow) is also associated.

### Table 6.3  Diffuse Reticular or Reticulonodular Disease

| Disease | Radiographic Findings | Comments |
| --- | --- | --- |
| **Lymphangitic carcinomatosis (e.g., from breast, lung, pancreas, stomach, thyroid, cervix and prostatic carcinoma) (Fig. 6.29)** | Usually uniform linear or reticular pattern with or without nodular component throughout both lungs but often more obvious in the lower-lung fields. Simulates interstitial pulmonary edema. Both hilar lymph node enlargement and pleural effusions are relatively common. Rapidly progressive loss of lung volume characteristic. | Caused by invasion of lymphatics from hematogenous metastases or, much less common, retrograde invasion into lungs from bronchopulmonary lymph nodes. Severe dyspnea is characteristic, which may even precede the radiographic manifestations. |
| **Lymphoma (Hodgkin's and non-Hodgkin's lymphoma) (Fig. 6.30)** | Interstitial infiltrate often most conspicuous in the perihilar area and usually associated with hilar and mediastinal lymphadenopathy, Pleural effusion may be present. | This pulmonary manifestation occurs probably by direct extension from hilar and mediastinal adenopathy. *Leukemia* and *macroglobutinemia Waldenström* can produce similar radiographic changes, but these are rare presentations in both disorders. |

*(continues on page 132)*

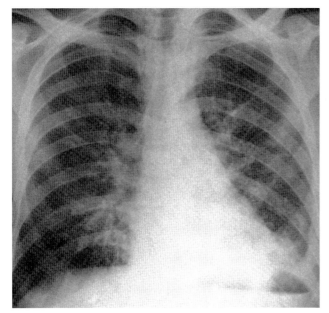

Fig. 6.**29 Lymphangitic carcinomatosis from gastric carcinoma.** Bilateral perihilar reticulonodular densities that are most prominent in the lower-lung fields are seen. Note also the left pleural effusion, whereas hilar lymph node enlargement cannot be appreciated in this case.

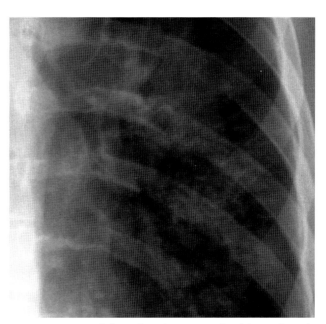

Fig. 6.**30 Non-Hodgkin's lymphoma.** Besides hilar and mediastinal lymph node enlargement, a reticular infiltrate In the left perihilar area is seen.

## Table 6.3  (Cont.) Diffuse Reticular or Reticulonodular Disease

| Disease | Radiographic Findings | Comments |
|---|---|---|
| **Pneumonias**<br>*Mycoplasma*<br>(Fig. 6.31) | Diffuse bilateral reticulonodular pattern, usually most conspicuous in lower lobes. | This presentation is less common than the localized form beginning with a fine reticular infiltrate that progresses rapidly to a consolidation. |
| **Influenza**<br>**Respiratory syncytial**<br>**virus (especially in**<br>**infants and young**<br>**children)**<br>**Rubeola (measles)**<br>**Varicella (Fig. 6.32)** | Mild increase in interstitial markings, particularly perihilar and at the bases to extensive reticulonodular involvement. Hilar lymph node enlargement occurs only in children. | Pulmonary findings in these viral infections similar to mycoplasma pneumonias. Localized or diffuse manifestations may progress to patchy consolidations. |
| **Cytomegalovirus**<br>(Fig. 6.33) | Reticulonodular pattern with nodules measuring up to 2 mm preferentially in periphery of middle and lower lobes. | This early-stage manifestation is followed by patchy consolidations. |
| **Pneumocystis carinii**<br>(Fig. 6.34) | Fine reticulonodular pattern particularly in perihilar areas. | This early-stage manifestation is followed by patchy consolidation simulating pulmonary edema. |
| **Atypical mycobacteria** (Fig. 6.35) | Multiple thin-walled cavities, preferentially located in the upper lobes, may produce a reticular pattern. Small nodules measuring lass than 1 cm may also be associated. | Radiographic presentation similiar to tuberculosis, but with a much greater tendency for cavitation. Usually found in patients with pre-existing pulmonary disease (e.g., emphysema and pneumoconiosis) or AIDS. |
| **Toxoplasmosis** | Reticular pattern that may be focal and indistinguishable from mycoplasma and viral pneumonia. Hilar lymph node enlargement is common. | Represents the early pulmonary manifestation of a generalized disease, |
| **Coccidioidomycosis**<br>**Blastomycosis**<br>**Cryptococcosis** | Disseminated, predominantly nodular disease that may progress to a reticulonodular pattern. | Rare presentation of these fungal diseases. |
| **Schistosomiasis** | Reticulonodular pattern, which can be associated with signs of pulmonary arterial hypertension (dilatation of pulmonary artery and its branches with rapid tapering toward periphery). | Interstitial changes produced by migration of ova through vessel wall with subsequent granuloma formation. Embolized ova can cause obliterative arteriolitis resulting in pulmonary hypertension. |
| **Filariasis**<br>(Fig. 6.36) | Fine reticular to reticulonodular pattern, often with nodules up to 5 mm, predominantly in mid and lower lung fields. Hilar lymph node enlargement can occur. | Disease confined to tropics *(tropical pulmonary eosinophilia)*. Patients with pulmonary disease do not usually have characteristic cutaneous and lymphatic changes such as elephantiasis. |

*(continues on page 134)*

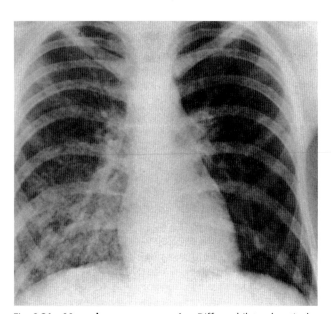

Fig. 6.**31** **Mycoplasma pneumonia.** Diffuse bilateral reticulonodular infiltrates are seen. The findings are most pronounced in the right lower lobe, where an early alveolar component is also present.

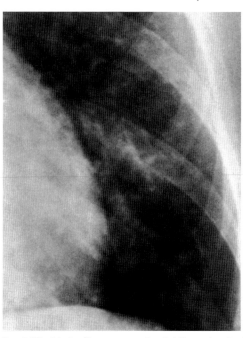

Fig. 6.**32** **Varicella pneumonia.** A bilateral reticulonodular infiltrate with numerous poorly defined nodules is predominantly involving the lower lobes, but only shown for the left side.

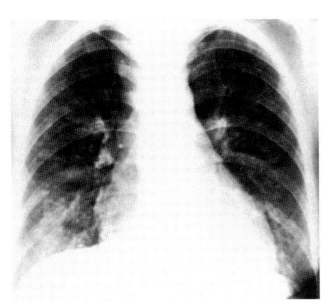

Fig. 6.**33** **Cytomegalovirus pneumonia** in patient with renal transplant. Reticulonodular and alveolar infiltrates are seen in both lower-lung fields.

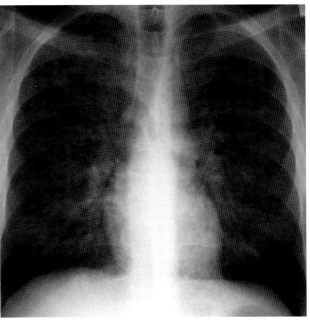

Fig. 6.**34** **Pneumocystis carinii pneumonia.** Extensive symmetrical reticulonodular infiltrates involving predominantly the perihilar areas are seen in this patient with AIDS.

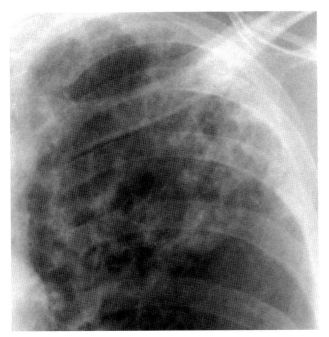

Fig. 6.**35** **Atypical mycobacterial infection.** Bilateral symmetrical reticulonodular to cystic infiltrates in the upper lobes are present in this patient with AIDS, but only shown for the left side.

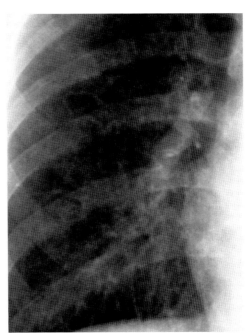

Fig. 6.**36** **Filariasis.** A fine reticuionodular pattern is seen in both lung fields, but only shown for the right side.

## Table 6.3   (Cont.) Diffuse Reticular or Reticulonodular Disease

| Disease | Radiographic Findings | Comments |
|---|---|---|
| Oily contrast material embolism (e.g., after lymphography) | Finely reticulogranular pattern caused by the oily contrast lodged in the terminal arterial branches. Rarely progresses to pulmonary edema. | Fat embolism after trauma, on the other hand, can only be diagnosed radiographically when the condition progresses to bilateral alveolar infiltrates with preferential involvement of the lung bases. |
| Interstitial edema (cardiogenic) | Increased interstitial markings, especially in the mid and lower lung fields, thickening of interlobular septa (Kerley A and B lines), loss of sharp definition of vascular structures, and perihilar haze, are characteristic. | Cardiomegaly (especially left atrial enlargement) and pulmonary venous hypertension (recognizable as redistribution of blood flow from the lower to the upper lobes) are usually present. |
| Fibrosis secondary to chronic left heart failure (Fig. 6.37) | Coarse, often poorly defined reticulation predominantly in mid and lower lung fields. | Results from recurrent episodes of interstitial and alveolar edema and hemorrhage. Differentiation between cardiogenic interstitial edema and fibrosis is often impossible on a single examination. |
| Acute bronchiolitis | Overinflation of the lungs is most characeristic. Often associated with reticulonodular densities with "miliary" appearance. | Viral (occasionally mycoplasma or bacterial) infection most commonly affecting children under 3 years of age and adults with pre-existing chronic respiratory disease. |
| Chronic bronchitis/ bronchiolitis (Fig. 6.38) | Coarse increase in interstitial markings often associated with some emphysema. | May also be referred to as "dirty chest". Bronchiectases may also be associated. |
| Bronchiolitis obliterans | Hyperinflation, often associated with reticulonodular pattern, especially in the lower lobes. | End stage of lower respiratory tract damage of a variety of diseases. |
| Bronchiolitis obliterans organizing pneumonia (BOOP) (Fig. 6.39) | Interstitial disease associated with patchy areas of consolidations that are commonly found bilaterally in the periphery of the mid and lower lung fields. | Clinically similar to idiopathic pulmonary fibrosis, but more responsive to steroid therapy and with better prognosis. |
| Cystic fibrosis (Fig. 6.40) | Coarse reticular pattern with cyst-like lesions often containing small air-fluid levels (bronchiectases). Overinflation is characteristically associated. Pulmonary fibrosis along the cardiac border may produce a "shaggy heart" sign. Recurrent pneumonias or atelectases are common. Signs of pulmonary arterial hypertension in the advanced stage. | Autosomal recessive transmission. Lack of pancreatic enzymes results in poor fat digestion and frequent small bowel obstructions (meconium ileus of the neonate). |
| Familial dysautonomia (Riley-Day syndrome) | Pulmonary findings indistinguishable from cystic fibrosis. | Autosomal recessive transmitted and almost exclusively found in Jews. Presents clinically with widespread neurologic disturbances. |
| Oxygen toxicity | "Spongy" lung caused by fibrosis, atelectasis and focal areas of emphysema. | Usually developing in premature infants receiving a high (up to 100%) percentage oxygen therapy for *respiratory distress syndrome* (hyaline membrane disease) or *Wilson-Mikity syndrome* (pulmonary dysmaturity). In the latter condition, similar radiographic findings are occasionally found before oxygen is given. Oxygen therapy in the adult may produce similar findings. |

*(continues on page 136)*

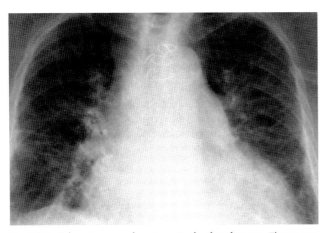

Fig. 6.**37**  **Fibrosis secondary to mitral valve disease.** The coarse and relatively poorly defined reticular pattern involving mainly the mid and lower lung fields persisted unchanged over a period of several years after mitral valve replacement.

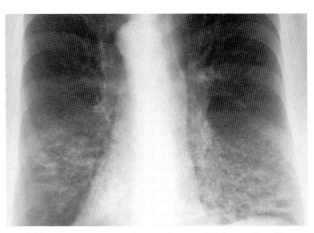

Fig. 6.**38**  **Kartagener syndrome (immotile/dysmotile cilia syndrome).** Situs inversus is associated with interstitial lung disease including bronchiectases mainly involving the lower lobes. Underdeveloped paranasal sinuses and sinusitis were also associated.

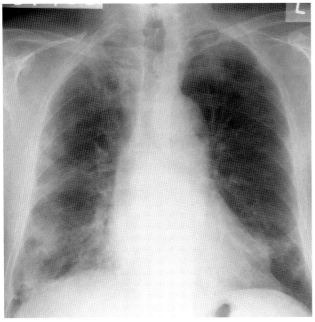

Fig. 6.**39**  **Bronchiolitis obliterans organizing pneumonia (BOOP).** Bilateral small nodular densities and patchy peripheral infiltrates are seen.

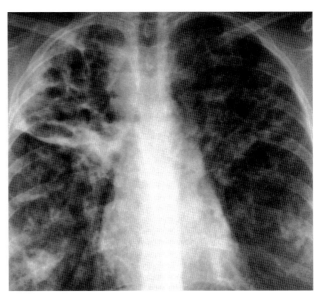

Fig. 6.**40**  **Cystic fibrosis.** A coarse reticulonodular pattern with cystic bronchiectases and fibroses is seen, involving predominantly the upper lobes. Note also the overinflated middle and lower lobes and the hilar prominence secondary to pulmonary arterial hypertension.

**Table 6.3 (Cont.) Diffuse Reticular or Reticulonodular Disease**

| Disease | Radiographic Findings | Comments |
|---|---|---|
| **Pneumoconiosis**<br>**Silicosis**<br>**(Fig. 6.41)** | Well-circumscribed nodular lesions ranging from 1 to 10 mm are usually the dominant radiographic feature, but are commonly associated with a reticular pattern that may even precede the nodules. Hilar lymph node enlargement is frequent, but the characteristic eggshell calcification occurs only in 5%. Progressive massive fibrosis (PMF) may develop in the upper lobes and present as bilateral homogenous opacifications that occasionally cavitate due to central ischemic necrosis or superimposed tuberculous caseation. | Exposure to highly concentrated silicon dioxide dust usually over 10 to 20 years before first radiographic manifestations.<br>*Caplan's syndrome:* association of necrobiotic (rheumatoid) nodules, ranging from 0.5 to 5 cm in diameter, rheumatoid arthritis, and silicosis. |
| **Coal miner's lung** | Radiographic findings similar to silicosis, although nodules are somewhat less well defined and hilar lymph node enlargement is less conspicuous. | Exposure to coal dust, which always contains small amounts of free silica but massive deposition of carbon, is assumed to be mainly responsible for the disease.<br>*Progressive massive fibrosis (PMF)* and *Caplan's syndrome* (association with necrobiotic lung nodules and rheumatoid arthritis) occur with even higher frequency than in silicosis. |
| **Asbestosis**<br>**(Fig. 6.42)** | Reticulonodular changes initially predominantly in lower lobes, later generalized. Pleural plaques with or without calcifications involving the parietal and diaphragmatic pleura are usually the dominant radiographic feature. Early interstitial changes combined with pleural thickening can produce "ground-glass" appearance. Conglomerate masses are occasionally found in an advanced stage and tend to show a lower zonal predominance. A combination of parenchymal and pleural changes may partially obscure the heart border ("shaggy heart" sign). Hilar lymph node enlargement does not occur. | Manifestations occur usually only 20 years after onset of exposure. Mesotheliomas and bronchogenic carcinomas are associated with a high incidence. |
| **Talcosis** | Pulmonary and pleural manifestations similar to asbestosis, but large opacities (conglomerate lesions) are more common. | Incidence of pleural and bronchogenic neoplasms also increased. |
| **Berylliosis** | Reticular to reticulonodular pattern with relatively poorly defined nodules that may calcify. Hilar lymph node enlargement occurs. Radiographic differentiation from sarcoidosis is usually not possible, unless the pulmonary nodules are calcified. Emphysematous changes, particularly in the upper lobe, result in a pneumothorax in 10%. | Berylliosis is not only found in workers exposed to beryllium (e.g., phosphorescent industry), but can also be attracted at home from contaminated work clothes or atmospheric pollution from a nearby plant. |
| **Aluminum (bauxite)**<br>**pneumoconiosis** | Reticular or reticulonodular pattern often associated with loss of lung volume and pleural thickening. Emphysematous bullae are common, resulting in a spontaneous pneumothorax. | Occurs a few months to several years of exposure in workers processing bauxite or inhaling fine aluminum powder. |
| **Pneumoconiosis caused by radiopaque dusts (iron [siderosis], tin [stannosis], barium [baritosis], antimony, and rare-earth compounds)** | Density of fine reticulonodular changes reflects atomic number and particle size of inhaled element. | Since these substances are not fibrogenic, no significant clinical symptoms are found in these pneumoconioses. |
| **Silo filler's disease**<br>**(NO$_2$ inhalation)**<br>**(Fig. 6.43)** | Bilateral reticulonodular infiltrates preferentially in the mid and lower lung fields that may progress rapidly to patchy alveolar densities and even massive pulmonary edema. | Pulmonary manifications resolve completely within a few days if not fatal. After an asymptomatic period of 2–5 weeks (second phase), the third phase of the disease becomes radiographically manifest as "miliary nodulation", representing bronchiolitis obliterans fibrosa. |

*(continues on page 138)*

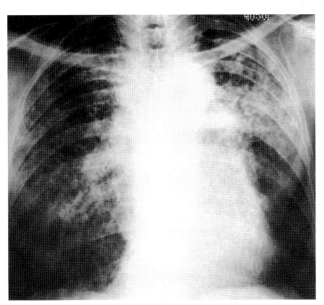

Fig. 6.**41** **Silicosis.** Fibrosis causing a reticulonodular pattern and honeycombing in the mid and upper lung fields and emphysematous changes at the bases are seen.

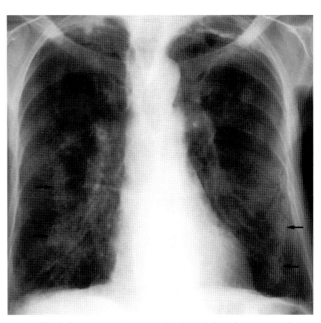

Fig. 6.**42** **Asbestosis.** Coarse reticulonodular changes and emphysema combined with pleural plaques and calcifications (arrows) are characteristic.

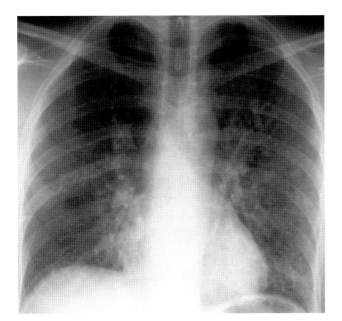

Fig. 6.**43** **Silo filler's disease.** Bilateral reticuionodular infiltrates with preferential involvement of the mid and lower lung fields are seen.

## Table 6.3 (Cont.) Diffuse Reticular or Reticulonodular Disease

| Disease | Radiographic Findings | Comments |
|---------|----------------------|----------|
| **Extrinsic allergic alveolitis due to organic dust (e.g., farmer's lung, bird-fancier's lung, mushroom-worker's lung, bagassosis [sugar cane], and others) (Fig. 6.44)** | Radiographic presentation ranges from diffuse poorly defined nodules, one to several millimeters in diameter and often associated with patchy infiltrates (acute stage) to coarse reticulation (chronic stage), Hilar lymph node enlargement is rare and never a dominant feature. | Clinical symptoms (dyspnea, often associated with dry cough and malaise) occur a few hours after exposure to relevant antigen. |
| **Drug-induced pulmonary disease (amiodarone, nitrofurantoin, busulphan, bleomycin, methotrexate, ganglionic blockers, and many others) (Figs. 6.45 and 6.46)** | Diffuse reticular to reticulonodular pattern, that might progress to patchy infiltrates and even pulmonary edema. | May be an allergic reaction to the drug, in which case it is associated with eosinophilia (e.g., nitrofurantoin), or a toxic effect causing interstitial infiltrates that may progress to fibrosis (e.g., chemotherapeutics). A variety of other drugs (e.g., penicillin, sulfonamides) cause a Loeffler's syndrome-like pattern. |
| **Connective tissue diseases (rheumatoid lung, scleroderma, systemic lupus erythematosus, dermatomyositis) (Fig. 6.47)** | Generalized reticular to reticulonodular disease, usually more prominent at the bases. Co-existing pleural effusion not common, except in lupus. | Pulmonary connective tissue manifestations of *polyarteritis nodosa* (another connective tissue disease) are highly variable and include increased interstitial markings, poorly defined nodules of varying size, and patchy consolidations. |

*(continues on page 140)*

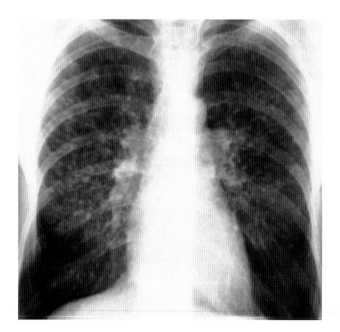

Fig. 6.**44 Farmer's lung.** A reticulonodular pattern is seen in both lungs with sparing of the bases and apices. The poorly defined nodules are indicative of the acute stage of the disease.

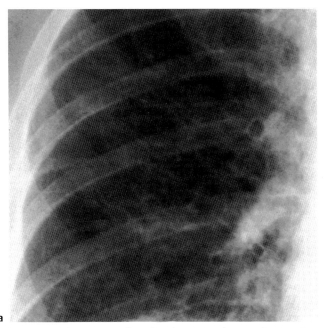

a

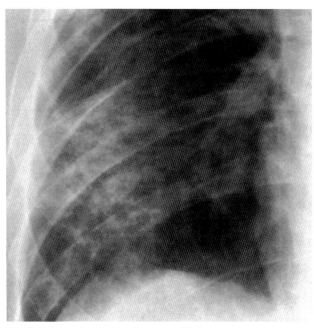

b

Fig. 6.**45   Bleomycin-induced pulmonary disease** (2 cases). **a** Early stage: Bilateral interstitial infiltrates of predominantly reticular nature are present, but only shown for the right mid and lower lung fields. **b** Advanced stage: Intestitial disease has progressed to patchy infiltrates.

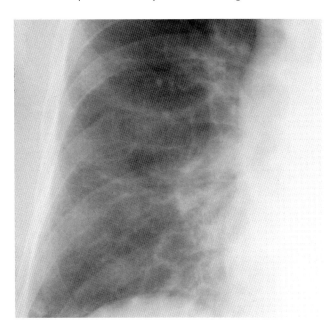

Fig. 6.**46   Amiodarone-induced pulmonary disease.** Bilateral interstitial and early alveolar infiltrates are present in the lower lung zones, but only shown for the right side.

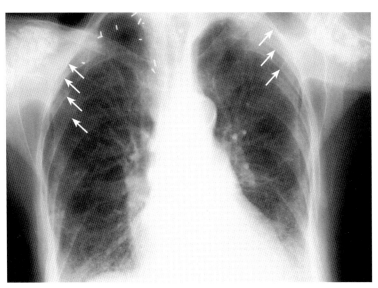

Fig. 6.**47   Scleroderma.** Interstitial lung disease with honeycombing at the lung bases is associated with extensive soft tissue calcifications in both shoulder regions and thinning of several ribs (arrows) in the upper chest bilaterally.

**Table 6.3    (Cont.) Diffuse Reticular or Reticulonodular Disease**

| Disease | Radiographic Findings | Comments |
|---|---|---|
| Sjögren's syndrome (Fig. 6.48) | Reticulonodular, similar to connective tissue disease. | Syndrome consists of keratoconjunctivitis sicca, xerostomia and recurrent parotid gland swelling. 90 % of the cases occur in women. |
| Idiopathic pulmonary hemosiderosis and Goodpasture's syndrome (Fig. 6.49) | Fine reticular pattern predominantly in mid- and lower-lung fields, found a few days after acute bleeding episode, evident as patchy consolidations. Persistence of a reticular to reticulonodular pattern after numerous bleeding episodes indicates irreversible interstitial changes resulting eventually in pulmonary fibrosis. Hilar enlargement and pleural effusions occur occasionally. | Clinical manifestations are repeated episodes of pulmonary hemorrhage resulting in anemia and pulmonary insufficiency. Goodpasture's syndrome additionally includes renal disease. Male predominance. |
| Langerhans cell histiocytosis (eosinophilic granuloma) (Fig. 6.50) | Poorly defined nodules up to 10 mm in diameter and fine reticular changes predominantly in the mid and upper lung fields. Disease may progress to honeycombing pattern. Hilar enlargement and pleural effusions are very rare and never a dominant feature. | Approximately one-third of patients are asymptomatic when initially diagnosed on a screening chest radiograph. Diagnosed most frequently in the 3rd and 4th decade with caucasian female predominance and often history of heavy cigarette smoking. |
| Sarcoidosis (Fig. 6.51) | Pulmonary manifestations vary from purely nodular to purely reticular, but a reticulonodular pattern is the most common presentation. Majority of cases is associated with significant hilar and mediastinal lymph node enlargement, which commonly precedes the lung involvement and may regress spontaneously in the presence of the latter. | Approximately half of patients are asymptomatic when first diagnosed on a screening chest radiograph. High incidence in black women living in the USA, usually diagnosed between 20 and 40 years of age. |
| Desquamative interstitial pneumonitis (DIP) (see Fig. 6.27) | Increased interstitial markings and reticulonodular densities, sometimes having a confluent or groundglass appearance are characteristic. Manifestations bilaterally symmetrical, and usually predominant in the lower lung fields, where they may cause a loss of definition of the vascular markings. | Etiology of DIP is unknown. May progress to pulmonary fibrosis (honeycombing) or regress spontaneously. *Lymphoid (LIP)* (Fig. 6.52) and *giant cell interstitial pneumonias (GIP)* are rare related conditions with similar radiographic features. |
| Idiopathic pulmonary fibrosis ("usual interstitial pneumonia" [UIP], Hamman-Rich syndrome) (Fig. 6.53) | Generalized coarse reticular or reticulonodular pattern. Honeycombing especially at the bases and loss of lung volume on serial films are often found. | Middle-aged and elderly men are most commonly affected. *Bronchiolitis obliterans with diffuse interstitial pneumonia (BIP)* represents a similar condition, but is associated with obliterating bronchiolitis. |
| Interstitial fibrosis secondary to pulmonary disease (Fig. 6.54) | Localized or generalized interstitial thickening. May be associated with fibrotic strands or scars. | Common cause of interstitial lung disease, though the offending agent is not always recognized. May be the sequela of recurrent infections, chronic aspiration, lung trauma, radiation, or thromboembolic disease (e.g., in sickle-cell anemia, where the lower lung fields are preferentially involved). |
| Familial and developmental disorders (tuberous sclerosis, lymphangiomyomatosis, neurofibromatosis, Gaucher's disease, Niemann-Pick disease, lipoid proteinosis) (Fig. 6.55) | Diffuse interstitial changes of a reticulonodular nature, with lower-lobe predilection. May progress to honeycombing and emphysema. | Associated findings on chest radiograph: Tuberous sclerosis: chylous effusions, osteoblastic lesions. Lymphangiomyomatosis: chylous effusions. Neurofibromatosis: skin nodules, scoliosis, rib notching, mediastinal masses. Gaucher's and Niemann-Pick disease: splenomegaly, osteopenia with compression fractures in vertebral bodies. Lipoid proteinosis: thickened vocal cords. |

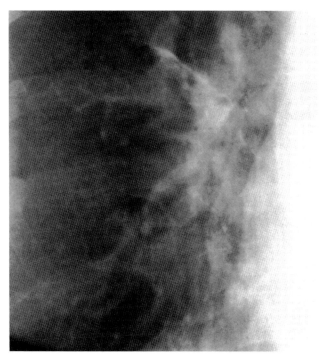

Fig. 6.**48** **Sjögren's syndrome.** Symmetrical reticulonodular infiltrates, predominantly involving the perihilar areas, but only shown for the right side.

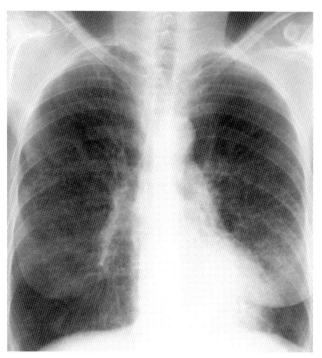

Fig. 6.**49** **Goodpasture's syndrome.** Bilateral interstitial disease of reticulonodular nature is seen mainly involving the mid and lower lung zones.

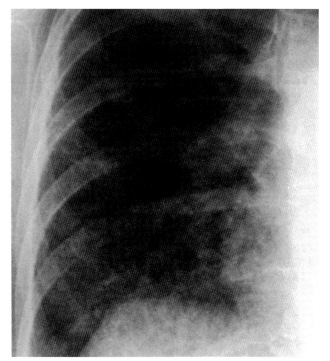

Fig. 6.**50** **Langerhans cell histiocytosis (eosinophilic granuloma).** Diffuse fine reticulonodular infiltrates with early honeycombing, involving both lungs symmetrically, but only shown for the right side.

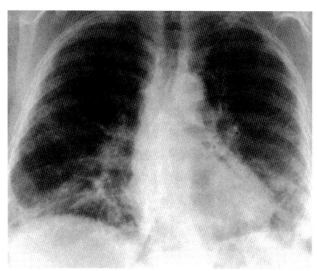

Fig. 6.**51** **Sarcoidosis.** Extensive bilateral reticulonodular disease with a few larger and poorly defined opacities at the bases is evident

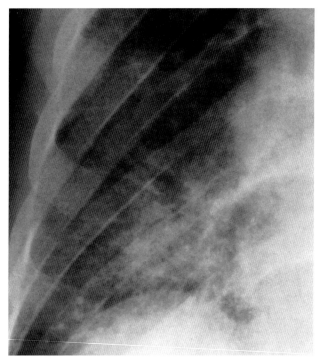

Fig. 6.**52    Lymphoid interstitial pneumonia (LIP).** Bilateral interstitial infiltrates in the mid and lower lung fields, with progression to consolidation in the central areas, are present, but only shown for the right lower lung field.

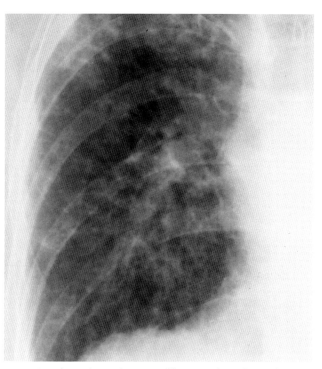

Fig. 6.**53    Idiopathic pulmonary fibrosis.** Bilateral reticulonodular disease with honeycombing is present, but only shown for the right side.

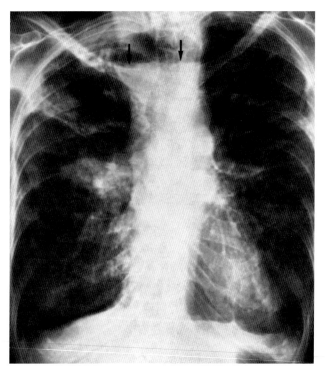

Fig. 6.**54    Chronic aspiration pneumonia in patient with Zenker diverticulum.** Diffuse coarse interstitial thickening is noted throughout both lung fields besides several areas of opacification resulting from more recent episodes of aspiration. Note also the large air-fluid level (arrows) in the Zenker diverticulum projecting just above the medial ends of both clavicles.

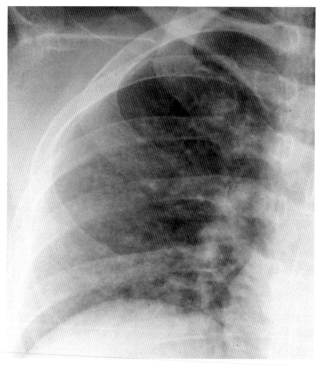

Fig. 6.**55    Tuberous sclerosis.** Bilateral interstitial lung disease of fine reticulonodular nature with beginning honeycombing at the bases is present, but only shown for the right side.

# 7 Pulmonary Edema and Symmetrical Bilateral Infiltrates

Pulmonary edema is caused by the accumulation of excessive fluid in both the interstitial and alveolar spaces. The two main factors responsible for the leak of fluid from the capillary space into the interstitial and subsequently the alveolar compartments are an *elevated capillary blood pressure* and *increased capillary permeability*. A decrease in either serum osmotic pressure or interstitial fluid pressure can contribute to the development of pulmonary edema, although these abnormalities are unlikely to cause edema by themselves. Other factors contributing to the development of pulmonary edema include a decrease in alveolar pressure and surface tension as well as obstruction of the lymphatics draining the lung interstitium, but their significance in this pathophysiologic mechanism is not clearly determined yet.

The most common cause of pulmonary edema resulting from an increased capillary pressure (*hydrostatic pulmonary edema*) is left ventricular failure (cardiogenic edema). Pulmonary veno-occlusive disease (e.g. idiopathic, congenital pulmonary vein anomalies, invasion or compression of pulmonary veins) may also induce hydrostatic pulmonary edema. An elevated pulmonary capillary pressure associated with a decreased serum osmotic pressure is responsible for pulmonary edema associated with renal failure and fluid overload. Neurogenic pulmonary edema results from a combination of both elevated capillary blood pressure and increased capillary permeability.

Pulmonary edema caused by increased capillary permeability is frequently referred to as *adult respiratory distress syndrome (ARDS)*. It is associated with sepsis, overwhelming pneumonia, aspiration, inhalation of noxious gases, pulmonary contusion, fractures (e.g. long bones and pelvis), near-drowning, burns, blood transfusions, major surgery (e.g. coronary bypass), prolonged hypotension, disseminated intravascular coagulation, and drug overdose.

Pulmonary edema is radiographically characterized by a bilateral, diffuse increase in interstitial markings with a loss of definition and by fluffy confluent opacities representing the alveolar process. This radiographic pattern is found most commonly in cardiogenic pulmonary edema, where the increased capillary blood pressure causes an abnormal plasma leak into the interstitial and alveolar spaces (Fig. 7.1). The edema accumulates predominantly in the most dependent portions of the lungs. In the upright position, this is in the mid- and, particularly, lower lung fields, whereas in the bedridden patient with the radiograph taken in the supine position, the edema appears more evenly distributed throughout both lungs. An unusual distribution pattern of the pulmonary edema might, however, be found with a pre-existing chronic lung disease (e.g. emphysema), where the edema spares the most severely damaged parts of the lungs (Fig. 7.2). Bronchogenic spread of various exogenous and endogenous materials and organisms may also cause diffuse alveolar infiltrates that may or may not be associated with interstitial disease. Finally, the infiltration of the alveolar and interstitial space with inflammatory or neoplastic cells can produce a radiographic appearance that also simulates pulmonary edema.

An unusual presentation of pulmonary edema takes the form of the *"bat's wing"* or *"butterfly pattern"*, in which the hilar and perihilar areas of the lungs are fairly dense and uniformly consolidated and the peripheral 2–3 cm of the lung parenchyma are relatively uninvolved (Fig. 7.3). This pattern

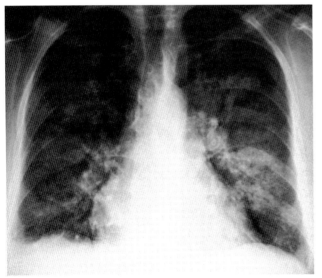

Fig. 7.1 **Cardiogenic pulmonary edema.** Cardiomegaly, bilateral interstitial and alveolar infiltrates involving predominantly the mid- and lower lung fields, and small pleural effusions are seen. This acute edema was caused by a left atrial myxoma that has suddenly enlarged secondary to intratumoral bleeding.

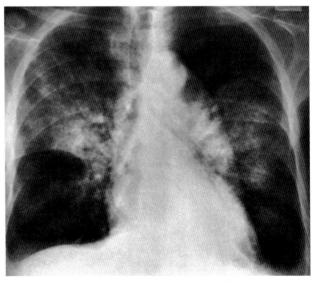

Fig. 7.2 **Cardiogenic pulmonary edema** in chronic obstructive pulmonary disease. Asymmetric distribution of the pulmonary edema that spares the parts of the lungs with the most severe emphysematous changes is seen.

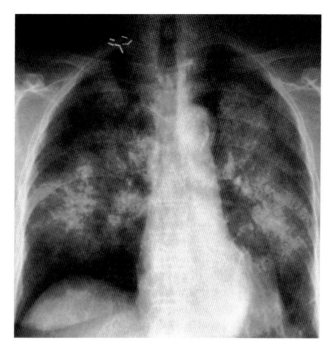

Fig. 7.**3**   **Pneumocystis carinii pneumonia** in compromised host. The pulmonary infiltrates, consisting of an interstitial (reticulonodular) and alveolar component, assume a *"bat's wing"* or *"butterfly pattern"*, sparing the peripheral 2–3 cm of the lung parenchyma.

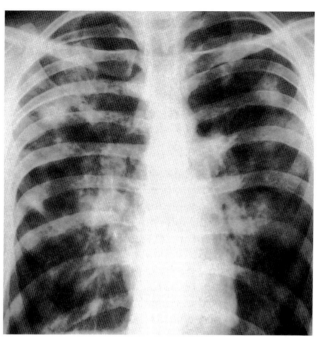

Fig. 7.**4**   **Loeffler's syndrome** (acute eosinophilic pneumonia). Bilateral patchy consolidations in the lung periphery parallel to the lateral chest wall are characteristic (*"reversed pulmonary edema pattern"*). The more central appearing infiltrates are anatomically located in the anterior or posterior lung periphery.

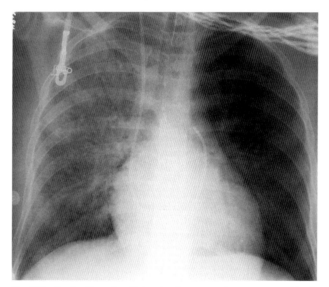

Fig. 7.**5**   **Aspiration.** A *unilateral pulmonary edema pattern* with air bronchograms is seen in the right lung. The aspiration occurred with the patient lying on his right side.

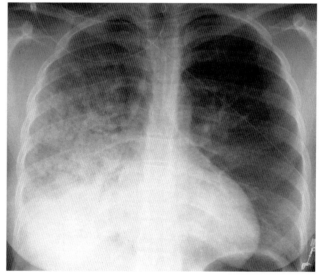

Fig. 7.**6**   **Narcotic abuse (cocaine).** Pulmonary edema is present bilaterally, but much more severe on the right side.

is relatively frequently seen with uremia, alveolar proteinosis, and pneumocystis carinii pneumonia, and with conditions causing pulmonary hemorrhage, such as idiopathic pulmonary hemosiderosis and polyarteritis nodosa. However, it is not at all pathognomonic of these conditions and can be found with virtually every disease known to produce a pulmonary edema pattern.

The *"reversed pulmonary edema pattern"* represents virtually a photographic negative of the "bat's wing" or "butterfly" pattern and is characterized by homogeneous consolidations in the lung periphery running more or less parallel to the lateral chest wall. This pattern is commonly found in acute (Loeffler's syndrome) and chronic eosinophilic pneumonia (Fig. 7.4).

An edema pattern caused by *pulmonary hemorrhage* frequently appears somewhat more dense than usual, although this finding largely depends on the employed radiographic technique. It may be observed with lung contusion, bleeding or clotting disorders, idiopathic pulmonary hemosiderosis, Goodpasture syndrome, systemic lupus erythematosus and chronic renal failure.

*Unilateral pulmonary edema* (Fig. 7.5 and 7.6) can be divided into ipsilateral and contralateral types. The former refers to conditions in which the pathogenetic mechanism

**Table 7.1  Pulmonary Edema and Symmetrical Bilateral Alveolar Infiltrates**

| Disease | Radiographic Findings | Comments |
|---|---|---|
| **Bronchioloalveolar carcinoma (alveolar cell carcinoma) (Fig. 7.7)** | Alveolar infiltrates combined with reticulonodular and linear densities. | Pleural effusions in approximately 10 %. Hilar and mediastinal lymph node enlargement uncommon. |
| **Lymphangitic carcinomatosis (Fig. 7.8)** | Interstitial and alveolar infiltrates similar to cardiogenic pulmonary edema, but with severe loss of lung volume and without cardiomegaly. Pleural effusions are commonly associated. | This represents an advanced stage of the disease that is virtually always associated with severe dyspnea. |

*(continues on page 146)*

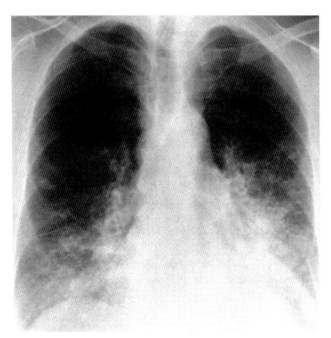

Fig. 7.**7**  **Bronchioloalveolar carcinoma.** Bilateral lower lobe infiltrates combined with poorly defined nodular densities are seen.

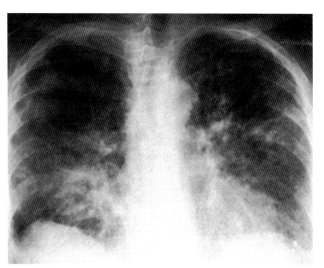

Fig. 7.**8**  **Lymphangitic carcinomatosis** from breast carcinoma (advanced stage). Mixed interstitial and alveolar pulmonary infiltrates with small pleural effusions are seen appearing similar to cardiogenic pulmonary edema. However, there is no cardiomegaly. Note also the marked loss of lung volume characteristically associated with advanced carcinomatosis.

leading to the asymmetry is on the side of the edema and include prolonged lateral decubitus position in cardiac decompensation, unilateral aspiration, pulmonary contusion, rapid thoracentesis, and unilateral bronchial or pulmonary venous obstruction. Contralateral pulmonary edema refers to accumulation of excess water in the normal lung opposite the diseased lung. The most common cause is chronic obstructive pulmonary disease (COPD), but it is also associated with acute pulmonary thromboembolism, Swyer-James syndrome, and unilateral lung destruction, fibrosis and pleural disease.

The differential diagnosis of pulmonary edema and of symmetrical bilateral alveolar infiltrates is discussed in Table 7.1. Occasionally an extensive diffuse interstitial disease simulates a pulmonary edema pattern when individual lesions, such as nodules, are so numerous that they become confluent and/or superimpose on each other while located in different planes. Therefore, the reader should also refer to Tables 6.1 and 6.2 of the preceding Chapter 6 for a complete differential diagnosis of a pulmonary edema pattern.

### Table 7.1 (Cont.) Pulmonary Edema and Symmetrical Bilateral Alveolar Infiltrates

| Disease | Radiographic Findings | Comments |
|---|---|---|
| Lymphoma and leukemia (Fig. 7.9) | Bilateral interstitial and alveolar infiltrates involving preferentially the perihilar areas and lower-lung fields. Appearance of symmetrical lung involvement may vary from predominantly interstitial edema to homogeneous consolidations. | In a lymphoma or leukemia patient these findings are, however, more often caused by intervening pneumonias, drug reaction, or hemorrhages, rather than by the underlying malignancy itself. |
| Kaposi's sarcoma (Fig. 7.10) | Numerous poorly defined metastases may mimic extensive bilateral infiltrates (opportunistic infections). | Common in male homosexual AIDS patients. |
| Pneumonia, bacterial (e.g., staphylococcus, Gram-negative bacteria, anaerobics, and tuberculosis) (Fig. 7.11) | Patchy confluent infiltrates often associated with areas of homogeneous consolidations. Cavitary lesions are relatively common and their demonstration is useful for the differentiation from other conditions presenting with a pulmonary edema pattern. | Bronchogenic spread by inhalation (e.g., staphylococcus), aspiration (e.g., anaerobic bacteria) or communication between abscess or cavity and bronchial system (e.g., tuberculosis). |
| Pneunomia, fungal (e.g., histoplasmosis, coccidioidomycosis, blastomycosis, aspergillosis, candidiasis) | Bilateral confluent infiltrates similar to aforementioned bacterial pneumonias, but cavitation less common. Hilar lymph node enlargement occurs only rarely, but when present, might be useful for differential diagnosis from nonfungal pneumonias. | This form is virtually limited to compromised hosts. An overwhelming exposure to the fungus rarely may produce this radiographic appearance in histoplasmosis. |
| Pneumonia, mycoplasma and viral (influenza, parainfluenza, coxsackie, adenovirus, psittacosis, varicella, SARS) (Fig. 7.12) | Diffuse reticular pattern with superimposed patchy alveolar infiltrates. Cavitation does not occur and hilar lymph node enlargement is extremely rare in the adult. | SARS (severe acute respiratory distress syndrome) presenting with a pulmonary edema pattern (15%) is associated with the highest mortality rate.<br><br>*Rickettsial infections* (e.g. Q-fever and Rocky Mountain spotted fever) may occasionally mimic viral pneumonias. |
| Cytomegalovirus (cytomegalic inclusion disease, CID) (Fig. 7.13) | Diffuse reticulonodular and alveolar infiltrates, preferentially involving the periphery of the middle and lower lobes. | In compromised hosts (e.g., renal transplants). |
| Pneumocystis carinii (Fig. 7.14) | Diffuse reticulonodular and alveolar infiltrates. Characteristically, the infiltrates are most pronounced in the perihilar areas, sparing the lung periphery. | Common presentation in compromised hosts and in the *acquired immune deficiency syndrome* (AIDS), where it is by far the most frequent complication. Despite certain differences in their characteristic locations, pneumocystis carinii and cytomegalovirus pneumonias can usually not be differentiated radiographically and, furthermore, often occur in the same patient. |

*(continues on page 148)*

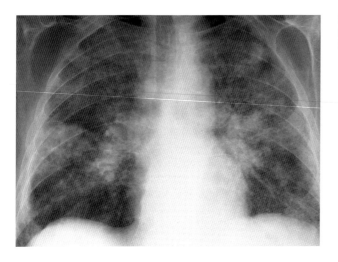

Fig. 7.**9** **Non-Hodgkin's lymphoma** (histiocytic). Bilateral interstitial and alveolar infiltrates are seen besides hilar and mediastinal lymph node enlargement.

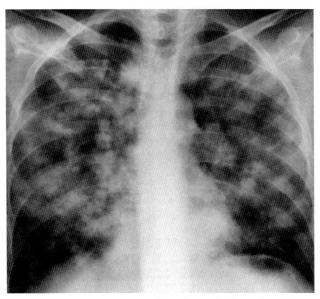

Fig. 7.**10**  **Kaposi's sarcoma.** Bilateral, poorly defined, confluent nodular densities are seen in this AIDS patient. Open lung biopsy revealed no evidence of an opportunistic infection.

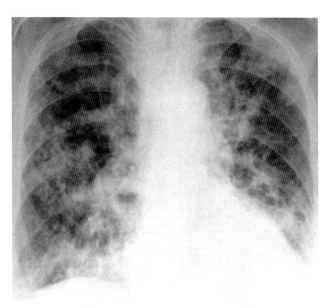

Fig. 7.**11**  **Pseudomonas pneumonia.** Extensive bilateral patchy infiltrates are seen.

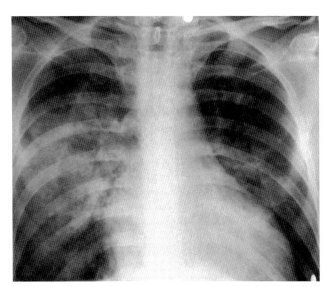

Fig. 7.**12**  **Influenza pneumonia.** Bilateral well defined airspace consolidations are seen, with considerably more extensive involvement of the right lung.

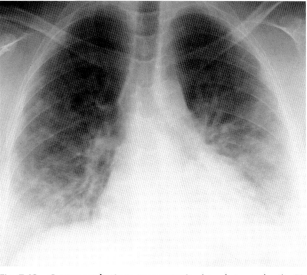

Fig. 7.**13**  **Cytomegalovirus pneumonia** (renal transplant). Bilateral reticulonodular and alveolar infiltrates, predominantly involving the mid and lower lung fields are evident.

Fig. 7.**14**  **Pneumocystis carinii pneumonia** (AIDS). Extensive bilateral reticulonodular interstitial disease is associated with early alveolar infiltrates with preferential perihilar and lower lung zone involvement.

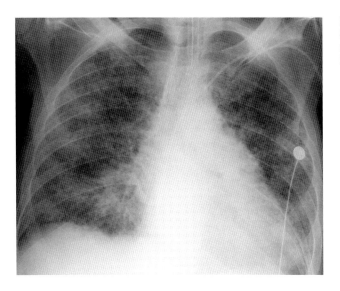

**Table 7.1 (Cont.) Pulmonary Edema and Symmetrical Bilateral Alveolar Infiltrates**

| Disease | Radiographic Findings | Comments |
|---|---|---|
| Malaria | Bilateral alveolar infiltrates. | Rare complication with Plasmodium falciparum in high blood concentrations. |
| Worm infestations (ascaris, strongyloidiasis, filariasis, paragonimiasis) | Bilateral confluent patchy infiltrates often with fine reticulonodular component. | Eosinophilia in peripheral blood invariably present in these conditions. |
| Oxygen therapy | Prolonged oxygen therapy in high concentration results in bilateral alveolar infiltrates (intra-alveolar hemorrhages) followed by hyaline membrane formation, and alveolar and interstitial fibroblastic proliferation. At this stage the bilateral infiltrates appear nonhomogeneous with "bubbly" appearance. | Similar process occurs in *premature infants* receiving oxygen therapy. A resembling radiographic appearance (diffuse bilateral infiltrates with "bubbly" appearance) may however, also be found in the *Wilson-Mikity syndrome* (pulmonary dysmaturity) of premature infants before oxygen therapy. *Transient tachypnea* of the newborn is caused by retained fetal lung fluid that clears rapidly in 1–4 days. |
| Noxious gas inhalation (e.g., silo filler's disease [nitrogen dioxide], or inhalation of carbon monoxide, smoke, and organophosphates [insecticides]) (Figs. 7.15 and 7.16) | Bilateral patchy parenchymal densities (transient pulmonary edema) developing within hours after exposure and clearing within a few days if not fatal. | This is the acute phase after exposure. Depending on the inhaled gas, other pulmonary complications such as atelectasis and pneumonic infiltrates can develop within days (e.g., in smoke inhalation) or weeks (e.g., in silofiller's disease, where a "miliary nodulation" pattern can be found). |
| Extrinsic allergic alveolitis (e.g., farmer's lung) | Bilateral reticulonodular pattern with poorly defined nodules and superimposed patchy, confluent infiltrates. | Develops within a few hours after exposure. |
| Berylliosis, acute | Diffuse confluent alveolar infiltrates. May be rapidly fatal. | Following overwhelming exposure to beryllium dust. |
| Aspiration of gastric content (Mendelson's syndrome) (Fig. 7.17) | Bilateral patchy infiltrates to homogeneous consolidations. Pulmonary distribution often asymmetric (depending on position of patient at time of aspiration). Resolves in 7–10 days with proper treatment (steroids and antibiotics). | Found with vomiting related to anesthesia, seizure, coma, alcohol and barbiturate poisoning. *Aspiration of hypertonic contrast agents* may cause pulmonary edema due to influx of fluid into the alveolar space. |
| Near-drowning (Fig. 7.18) | Symmetrical pulmonary edema that may occasionally be delayed for up to 2 days. Resolution occurs usually in 3–5 days, but may only be complete in 10 days. | There is radiographically no difference between fresh and saltwater aspiration. |
| Fluid overload/ overtransfusion (hypervolemia, hypoproteinemia) | Bilateral patchy infiltrates. Rapidly clearing with appropriate treatment. | Pulmonary edema also may be the result of an *incompatible blood transfusion*. |

*(continues on page 150)*

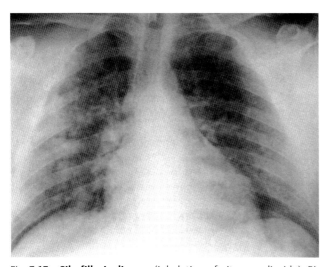

Fig. 7.**15**  **Silo filler's disease** (inhalation of nitrogen dioxide). Bilateral patchy infiltrates are seen throughout both lungs.

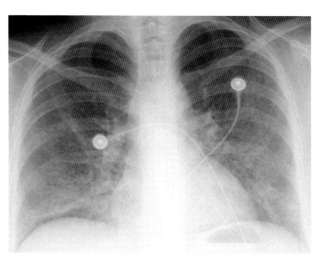

Fig. 7.**16**  **Smoke inhalation.** Early interstitial and alveolar edema is seen bilaterally in the mid and lower lung zones.

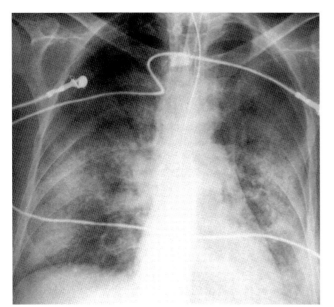

Fig. 7.**17**  **Aspiration** in an alcoholic (Mendelson's syndrome). Extensive bilateral alveolar infiltrates producing homogeneous consolidations with air bronchograms are seen.

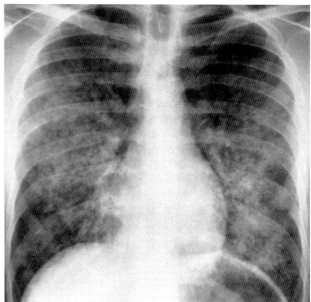

Fig. 7.**18**  **Near-drowning** in fresh water. Pulmonary edema developed 12 hours after admission. The initial radiograph performed at the time of admission was essentially negative.

## Table 7.1 (Cont.) Pulmonary Edema and Symmetrical Bilateral Alveolar Infiltrates

| Disease | Radiographic Findings | Comments |
|---|---|---|
| Narcotic abuse (Fig. 7.19) | Bilateral patchy densities to massive confluent consolidations. May be delayed up to 10 hours after admission and resolves rapidly within 1 to 2 days. | Most often a complication of heroin or methadone overdose. If the edema pattern persists after 2 days, aspiration or superimposed bacterial pneumonia should be suspected. |
| Drug-induced pulmonary disease (Fig. 7.20) | Pulmonary manifestations vary from minimal interstitial disease to patchy consolidations and massive pulmonary edema. The time required for both the development and resolution of the pulmonary disease depends on the mechanism involved and is extremely variable, ranging from a few minutes to several months. Resolution may not always be complete. | Pulmonary disease is caused by either drug hypersensitivity or drug toxicity. The following manifestations can be found: spasmodic asthma, noncardiogenic edema, hypersensitivity pneumonitis with or without peripheral eosinophilia, interstitial and alveolar pneumonitis, systemic lupus erythematosus, and pulmonary vasculitis. |
| Adult respiratory distress syndrome (ARDS) (Fig. 7.21) | Bilateral alveolar pulmonary infiltrates characteristically delayed up to 12 hours after clinical onset of respiratory failure. May progress to extensive bilateral consolidations within 48 hours. Absence of pleural effusions is characteristic. Interstitial emphysema, pneumomediastinum, and pneumothorax can result from positive pressure ventilation. Slow resolution begins after one week, when the infiltrates become inhomogeneous and demonstrate a reticular and cystic component (DD: superimposed pneumonia with microabscesses). | Mechanisms of lung capillary leak resulting in ARDS are not clear. Hypovolemic shock plays an important role, but other factors (e.g., endotoxins, vasoactive agents) must be involved also. ARDS has been associated with sepsis, disseminated intravascular coagulation (DIC), vasoactive substance released from traumatized tissue or blood constituents, prolonged respirator care and cardiopulmonary bypass.<br>*Respiratory distress syndrome (hyaline membrane disease)* in infants is characterized by overinflated lungs with granular appearance, air bronchograms, interstitial pulmonary emphysema, and atelectatic areas. |
| Disseminated intravascular coagulation (DIC) (Fig. 7.22) | Minimal scattered parenchymal densities to massive pulmonary edema. In the latter case, both pulmonary manifestations and the course of the disease are indistinguishable from the adult respiratory distress syndrome. | Refers to uncontrolled clotting within blood vessels resulting in coagulation failure due to fibrinogen deficiency, thrombocytopenia and excessive fibrinolysis ("consumption coagulopathy"). Always secondary to another disorder such as shock, sepsis, cancer, obstetric complications, burns, and liver disease. |

*(continues on page 152)*

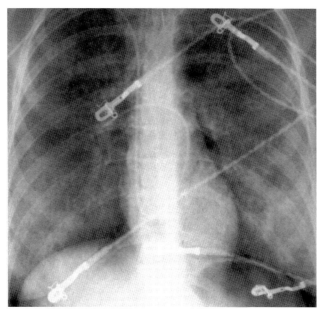

Fig. 7.**19    Drug abuse (heroin).** Diffuse bilateral opacification of the lungs with confluent alveolar infiltrates is seen.

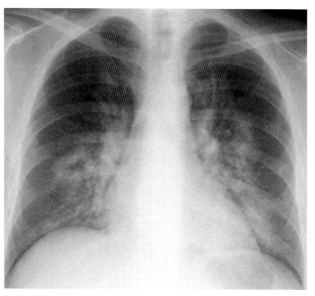

Fig. 7.**20    Drug-induced pulmonary disease** (methotrexate). Bilateral patchy perihilar infiltrates are seen.

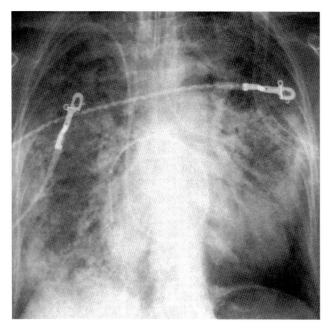

Fig. 7.**21    Adult respiratory distress syndrome** (ARDS). Extensive bilateral consolidations with air bronchograms and scattered cystic radiolucencies are seen in this patient one week after episode of severe hemorrhagic shock.

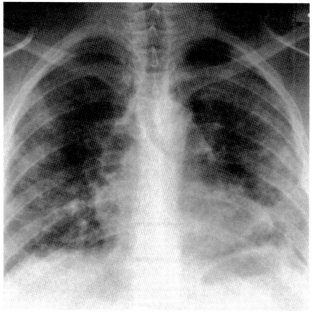

Fig. 7.**22    Disseminated intravascular coagulation** (DIC). Symmetric bilateral patchy densities are seen in this patient with septic abortion.

## Table 7.1 (Cont.) Pulmonary Edema and Symmetrical Bilateral Alveolar Infiltrates

| Disease | Radiographic Findings | Comments |
|---|---|---|
| Pulmonary contusion (Fig. 7.23) | Parenchymal densities caused by hemorrhages are seldom symmetrical (involvement is greater on the side of maximum impact, that may be evident by rib fractures). In contrast to fat embolism, hemorrhages are invariably apparent within the first 6 hours and resolve rapidly within one week. | Most common complication of blunt chest trauma. |
| Pulmonary hemorrhage, nontraumatic (e.g., bleeding-diathesis, idiopathic pulmonary hemosiderosis, Goodpasture's syndrome, polyarteritis nodosa, Wegener's granulomatosis) (Fig. 7.24) | Bilateral alveolar infiltrates clearing within 2 to 3 days after single bleeding episode. Reticular changes may, however, persist for several more days in these areas, especially in idiopathic pulmonary hemosiderosis and Goodpasture's syndrome. | Pulmonary hemorrhage in idiopathic pulmonary hemosiderosis, Goodpasture's syndrome, polyarteritis nodosa, and Wegener's granulomatosis is caused by severe damage to the alveolar-capillary membranes secondary to an alteration in the immune system. Hemorrhagic pulmonary edema based on a similar mechanism also can be found in *acute glomerulonephritis*. |
| Thromboembolic disease (Fig. 7.25) | Bilateral consolidations preferentially in lower lobes. Associated findings include enlarged hilar arteries with abrupt peripheral tapering, pulmonary oligemia (Westermark sign), loss of lung volume (elevated diaphragms), small pleural effusions, and prominent azygos vein. | This is a rare pulmonary manifestation of extensive thromboembolism with infarction. The radiographic findings usually are rather minimal considering the severity of clinical symptoms. |
| Fat embolism (Fig. 7.26) | Bilateral peripheral alveolar infiltrates that predominantly involve the lower lung fields. Usually only apparent 1–2 days after trauma. Resolution requires 1 week or longer. Absence of cardiomegaly, pulmonary venous hypertension, and interstitial edema differentiates this condition from cardiogenic edema. | Fat embolism after trauma goes unrecognized in the majority of cases because of mild clinical symptoms and minimal radiographic changes. However, the presence of petechial skin rash and cerebral pathology together with the described radiographic lung manifestations is virtually diagnostic. *Oily contrast material embolism* (e.g. after lymphography) progresses only exceptionally to this stage. |
| Amniotic fluid embolism | Widespread pulmonary consolidations, often rapidly fatal | Predisposing factors include tumultuous labor, intrauterine fetal death, old age of mother, and multiparity. Pathogenesis derives from 3 factors associated with the entrance of amniotic fluid into the maternal circulation: 1 embolic obstruction of pulmonary vasculature by particulate matter in the amniotic fluid, 2 anaphylactoid reaction to particulate matter in the amniotic fluid, and 3 coagulation failure secondary to disseminated intravascular coagulation (DIC). |

*(continues on page 154)*

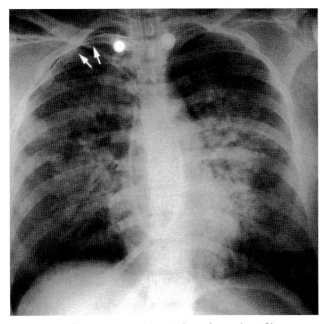

Fig. 7.**23** **Pulmonary contusion.** Bilateral, patchy infiltrates are present. A small right apical pneumothorax is also present (arrows).

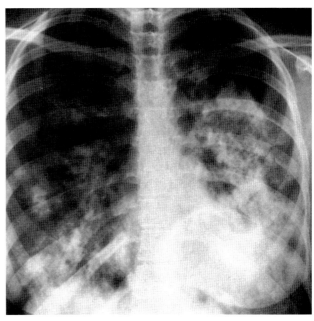

Fig. 7.**24** **Goodpasture's syndrome.** Bilateral, patchy and largely confluent infiltrates are seen in the mid and lower lung fields.

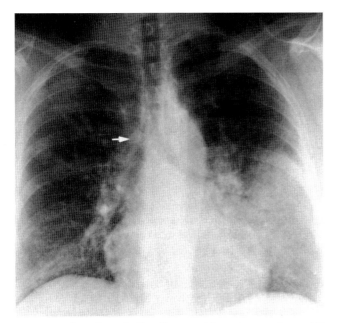

Fig. 7.**25** **Thromboembolic disease.** Bilateral, prominent hili (pulmonary arteries) and perihilar densities are seen. The area of consolidation along the left chest wall proved to be a large infarct. Note also the distended azygos vein (arrow).

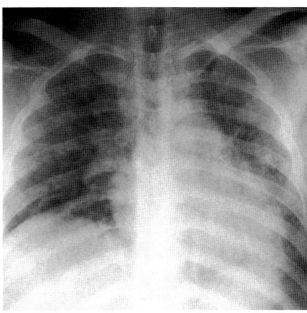

Fig. 7.**26** **Fat embolism.** Bilateral patchy alveolar infiltrates that are confluent in many areas are seen.

## Table 7.1 (Cont.) Pulmonary Edema and Symmetrical Bilateral Alveolar Infiltrates

| Disease | Radiographic Findings | Comments |
|---|---|---|
| Neurogenic disorders (e.g., head trauma, seizures, increased intracranial pressure) (Fig. 7.27) | Edema is frequently asymmetric. Resolution occurs within several days following surgical relief of increased intracranial pressure. | Related to increased intracranial pressure, but mechanism is not clear. May be caused by the combination of increased capillary pressure and abnormal capillary permeability in both lungs. |
| Cardiovascular disease causing pulmonary venous hypertension (see Figs. 7.1 and 7.2) | Bilateral, symmetrical, interstitial and alveolar densities are the usual presentation. May be preceded by a predominantly interstitial phase with Kerley A and B lines. Pulmonary venous hypertension, evident by redistribution of blood flow from the lower to upper lung fields almost invariably present. Cardiomegaly is usually present if the edema is caused by left heart failure.<br>An asymmetric edema pattern can be found in emphysema, where the edema spares the most severely damaged parts of the lung. A more unilateral distribution is observed in patients lying preferentially on one side. | Most common cause of the pulmonary edema pattern. Cardiogenic causes include left ventricular failure, mitral valve disease, left atrial myxoma, cor triatriatum and hypoplastic left heart syndromes. Noncardiogenic causes include partial occlusion of the pulmonary veins by thrombosis, fibrosis or tumor, and an anomalous pulmonary venous return. Impairment of the lymphatic drainage of the lung interstitium may also contribute to the development of pulmonary edema. |
| Renal failure/uremia (Fig. 7.28) | Bilateral symmetrical infiltrates similar to cardiogenic pulmonary edema, but may show "butterfly pattern" and can appear quite dense. | The occasionally observed greater radiographic density of the pulmonary edema in renal failure can be explained by the fibrogeneous nature of the edema with hemorrhage, cellular infiltration, and organization ("uremic pneumonia"). Calcification of the underlying lung parenchyma can also contribute to the overall increased density of the edema in chronic renal failure (Fig. 7.29). |
| Radiation pneumonitis | Infiltrates confined to areas of irradiation. | Lung manifestations usually begin to appear 1–6 months after cessation of treatment. |
| High altitude | Patchy, irregular pulmonary edema. Rapid clearing after oxygen administration or return to lower altitude. | Symptoms develop between 12 hours to 3 days after arrival at high altitude (3500 m above sea level and higher). |
| Rapid lung re-expansion | Unilateral, unless both lungs are re-expanded. | Following thoracentesis of a large (50% and more) pneumothorax or hydrothorax that has been present for several days. |
| Alveolar proteinosis (Fig. 7.30) | Bilateral confluent alveolar infiltrates, often with "butterfly distribution". Very slow and often asymmetric progression or resolution of infiltrates is characteristic. Fatal in approximately one-third of cases. | Predominantly in men between 20 and 50 years of age. Patients susceptible to opportunistic fungal infections, especially nocardiosis. |
| Alveolar microlithiasis (see Fig. 6.18) | Superimposition and summation of discrete and extremely sharply defined microliths measuring less than 1 mm diameter produce symmetrical bilateral opacification that is usually most pronounced in the lower lung fields. | Rare disorder of obscure etiology with familial occurrence in over 50%. Usually found in patients under the age of 50, but may already be observed in infants. |
| Sarcoidosis | A predominantly alveolar pattern is extremely rare, more often it is mixed with a reticulonodular component. | Hilar and mediastinal lymph node enlargement is often present. |

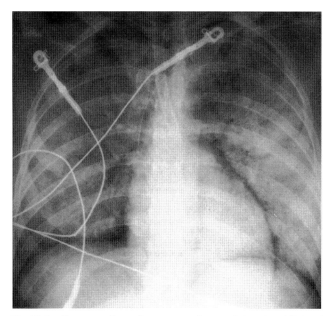

Fig. 7.**27** **Neurogenic pulmonary edema.** Extensive bilateral opacification of both lungs, that is denser on the left than right side, is caused by alveolar pulmonary edema. Note also that the tip of the endotracheal tube has been placed erroneously in the left main bronchus.

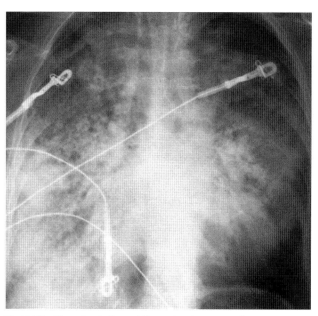

Fig. 7.**28** **Uremia.** A dense bilateral pulmonary edema pattern is seen.

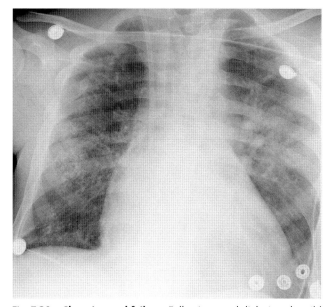

Fig. 7.**29** **Chronic renal failure.** Following renal dialysis only mild pulmonary edema in the left perihilar area is present. The sharply demarcated punctate and reticular opacities in the right lung sparing its periphery are caused by extensive parenchymal calcifications.

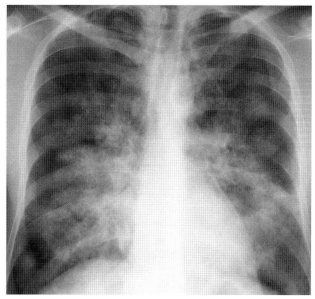

Fig. 7.**30** **Alveolar proteinosis.** Bilateral patchy and confluent alveolar infiltrates sparing the lung periphery ("butterfly pattern") is seen. Characteristic is a slow progression and resolution of the infiltrates over months.

# 8 Pulmonary Nodules and Mass Lesions

A variety of lesions located outside the lung parenchyma can simulate pulmonary nodules and mass lesions. Extrapulmonary lesions projecting into the lung fields and simulating intrapulmonary conditions are either surrounded by air (e.g., skin lesions) or have a density that is significantly greater than that of the surrounding soft tissue. The latter is the case, for example, in calcified and ossified lesions.

*Nipple shadows* frequently simulate pulmonary coin lesions on the frontal chest radiograph but can be differentiated from them easily by repeating the chest radiograph with arms elevated over the head. With the latter technique, it is possible to separate a nipple shadow that by chance was superimposed on a true intrapulmonary nodule. Similarly, skin tumors (e.g., *neurofibromas*) must be differentiated from intrapulmonary mass lesions (Fig. 8.1 and 8.2). When skin tumors are multiple, some of them are likely to project outside the lung fields, thus facilitating the correct diagnosis. Focal rib lesions can be diagnosed by confirming with oblique views that the lesion cannot be seen separately from the bone in different projections. Cloth and film artifacts must also be excluded.

Pleural and extrapleural mass lesions protruding into the lung can be difficult to differentiate from a pulmonary lesion abutting the visceral pleura. When the lesions are seen tangentially, both pleural and extrapleural lesions are said to form an obtuse angle with the chest wall.

However, pulmonary mass lesions abutting the pleural surface (e.g., "Hampton's hump" in pulmonary infarction) may also form an obtuse angle. Furthermore, larger pleural and extrapleural lesions often resemble the shape of a female breast when viewed in profile. In these cases an obtuse angle with the chest wall is found only on the upper margin of the lesion, whereas it becomes acute on its lower end. Pleural and extrapleural lesions, therefore, can be more reliably differentiated from pulmonary lesions by demonstrating a triangular soft-tissue density at the side where the lesion blends into the chest wall (Fig. 8.3). This triangular soft-tissue density is caused by gradual separation of the pleura from the chest wall by the mass lesion. Demonstration of this sign requires viewing the lesion in profile. It cannot be seen when a tumor originates from the visceral pleura and grows exclusively into the lung parenchyma. It might be hidden at the inferior margin of the breast-shaped pleural or extrapleural lesion.

Pleural and extrapleural lesions usually have a well-demarcated surface when projected in profile, since they are covered with pleura, whereas pulmonary lesions may have smooth or shaggy margins. Since pleural and extrapleural lesions often have a long, flat appearance, they may only produce a vague and indistinct increase in the lung density when seen en face. Pleural lesions are often lobulated or multiple, whereas extrapleural lesions are often associated with a rib fracture or rib destruction.

Mass lesions and loculated pleural effusions within the interlobar fissures must also be differentiated from parenchymal lung lesions. This is usually possible because of the

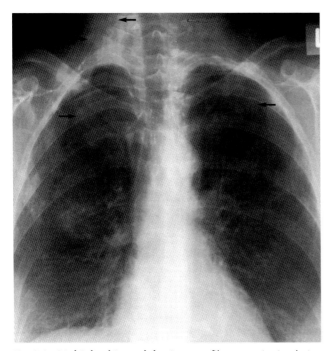

Fig. 8.**1 Multiple skin nodules** in neurofibromatosis simulating intrapulmonary nodules. Multiple nodular lesions (arrows) are seen. Some of them are projecting into the lung fields, while others are clearly outside the lungs.

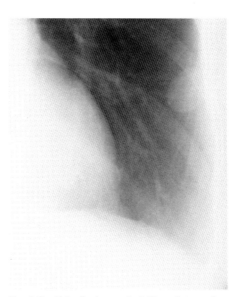

Fig. 8.**2 Skin lesion mimicking intrapulmonary nodule.** An ovoid density projects into the left lower lung field.

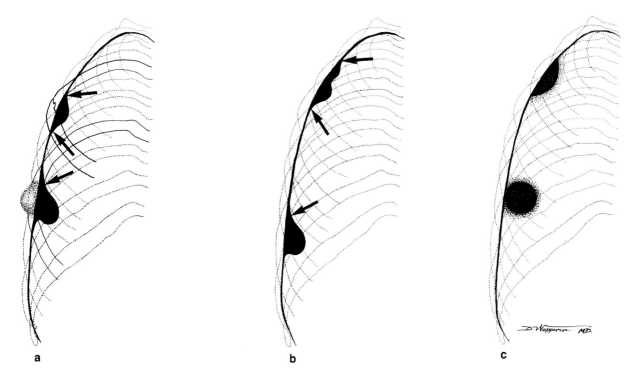

Fig. 8.**3** **Differential diagnosis of a extrapleural, b pleural, and c pulmonary lesions**, when seen in profile. **a** Extrapleural lesions are often associated with rib lesions (fracture or destruction) and lift up the parietal and visceral pleurae from the chest wall, which is evident as a triangular density at the upper and lower margin of the lesion (arrows). **b** Pleural lesions are often lobulated and also demonstrate the "pleural lift-up sign" at their margins (arrows), unless they originate from the visceral pleura and grow primarily into the lung parenchyma, **c** Pulmonary lesions abutting the pleural surface do not separate the pleura from the chest wall and may be well or poorly demarcated. An acute angle between a lesion and the chest wall at both its superior and inferior margins is also characteristic of a pulmonary mass. See text for more detailed discussion.

characteristic anatomic location, oblong shape, and well-defined margins of such pleural lesions. When viewed tangentially their ends blend imperceptibly with the corresponding interlobar fissure.

The *margins of true pulmonary nodules* may be smooth, lobulated or spiculated. In general, smooth margins suggest benignity and spiculation malignancy, whereas lobulation is found with approximately equal frequency in benign and malignant lesions. *Satellite lesions* are defined as small nodu-lar opacities in close proximity to a larger, usually solitary lesion. They usually indicate an infectious etiology such as a tuberculoma.

The differential diagnosis of solitary or multiple pulmonary nodules and masses is summarized in Table 8.**1**, while the differential diagnosis of disseminated pulmonary nodules measuring less than 1 cm in diameter has already been summarized in Table 6.**1** of chapter **6**.

**Table 8.1 Pulmonary Nodules and Mass Lesions**

| Disease | Radiographic Findings | Comments |
|---|---|---|
| **Bronchogenic cyst** (Fig. 8.4) | Solitary, sharply circumscribed, round mass measuring up to several centimeters in diameter, most commonly in the medial third of the lungs with predilection for lower lobes. Cavitation occurs with infection, resulting in communication with the bronchial system. Calcification of cyst wall and cyst content is very rare. | Approximately two-thirds of bronchogenic cysts are pulmonary and the rest mediastinal in origin. Congenital and acquired (e.g., following lung abscess or trauma) cysts are radiographically indistinguishable from each other. Acquired cysts have no site predilection. |
| **Intralobar bronchopulmonary sequestration** (Fig. 8.5) | Well-defined, homogeneous mass usually contiguous with the diaphragm and characteristically located in the posterobasal segment of a lower lobe (left to right ratio, 3 : 1), whereas the upper lobes are rarely affected. Air-fluid levels are seen within the lesion when communication with the bronchial system occurs, usually because of infection. Angiographically, large feeding arteries from the thoracic and/or abdominal aorta are characteristic. Drains to pulmonary veins. | Asymptomatic until sequestered tissue becomes infected. This often occurs only in adulthood, when the anomaly is usually first recognized. *Congenital cystic adenomatoid malformation* (type III) may also present as large bulky mass (see Fig. 9.**7**). |

*(continues on page 160)*

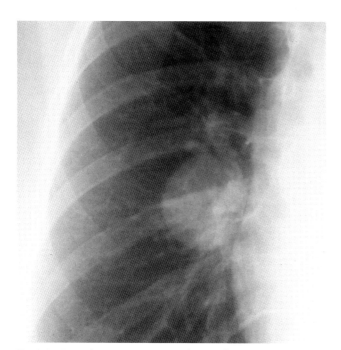

**Fig. 8.4 Bronchogenic cyst.** A solitary, sharply circumscribed round lesion projects into the right hilum.

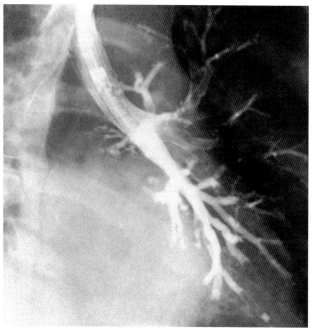

**Fig. 8.5 Intralobar bronchopulmonary sequestration.** A homogeneous mass contiguous to the diaphragm is seen in the left lower lobe displacing the opacified bronchi laterally (bronchography).

**Table 8.1  (Cont.) Pulmonary Nodules and Mass Lesions**

| Disease | Radiographic Findings | Comments |
|---|---|---|
| **Extralobar bronchopulmonary sequestration (Fig. 8.6)** | Well-defined homogeneous mass that is related to the left diaphragm (above or below) in 90 % of patients, and in the remaining cases related to the right diaphragm or the mediastinum. Cavitation is rare, since the lesion is enclosed by its own visceral pleura. Blood supply derives from a systemic artery (usually from the abdominal aorta or one of its branches) and drainage occurs via the inferior vena cava, the azygos or hemiazygos system, or the portal vein. | Frequently associated with other more severe congenital anomalies (e.g. diaphragmatic hernias, eventrations and foregut communications), which may result in death during infancy. |
| **Arteriovenous fistulas (Fig. 8.7)** | Solitary or less common, multiple, well-defined round or slightly lobulated lesion(s) measuring up to several centimeters. Change in size and shape with Vasalva and Mueller maneuvers. Predilection for medial third of lungs and lower lobes. Feeding artery and/or draining vein can often be identified as band-like density extending from hilum to lesion. Calcifications (phleboliths) are rarely seen. | Approximately half of the cases are associated with *hereditary hemorrhagic telangiectasia (Rendu-Osler-Weber disease)* with arteriovenous fistulas in the skin, mucous membranes, and other organs. A *pulmonary artery branch aneurysm* (Fig. 8.**8**) can also present as a central pulmonary nodular lesion. |
| **Pulmonary vein varicosity** | One to several round, well-defined densities measuring up to a few centimeters in diameter. Characteristic central location, best seen on lateral radiograph projecting posterior and inferior to the hilar structures. Change shape and size with Valsalva and Mueller maneuvers (similar to arteriovenous fistulas). | Congenital or acquired tortuosity and dilatation of a pulmonary vein just before its entrance into the left atrium. |
| **Bronchial adenoma (Fig. 8.9 and 29.10)** | Twenty percent present as solitary, well-circumscribed and often slightly lobulated peripheral lung lesions measuring usually 1 to 3 cm (occasionally up to 10 cm) in diameter. Calcifications/ossifications are rarely visible on chest radiographs, but may be identified on CT in about 30 % of cases. Eighty percent are centrally located in the bronchial lumen presenting with segmental or lobar atelectasis and obstructive pneumonia. Cavitation is extremely rare. Hilar, mediastinal and bony metastases (lytic and/or blastic) are occasionally associated. | Locally invasive, low-grade malignant tumors with tendency for recurrence and occasional metastases to extrathoracic sites. Four types: carcinoid (90 %), cylindroma (6 %), mucoepidermoid carcinoma (3 %) and pleomorphic adenoma (1 %). Age ranges from 12 to 60 years (mean age 35 to 45 years) without sex predilection, but very rare in blacks. Clinical manifestations include hemoptysis (50 %), atypical asthma, persistent cough and recurrent obstructive pneumonia. |

*(continues on page 162)*

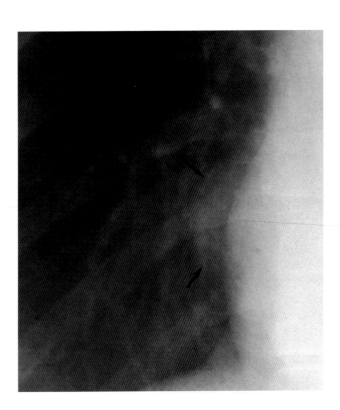

Fig. 8.**6  Extralobar bronchopulmonary sequestration.** A well-defined mass (arrows) is seen abutting the right border of the mediastinum posterior to the heart.

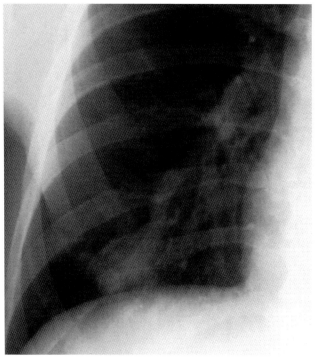

Fig. 8.**7 Arteriovenous fistula.** A slightly lobulated mass that is connected with the hilum by a bandlike density (feeding artery) is seen in the right lower lobe.

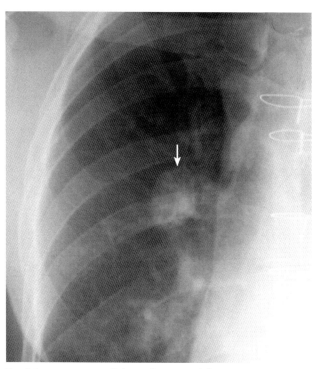

Fig. 8.**8 Aneurysm of the right upper lobe artery in Behçet's syndrome.** A nodular lesion (arrow) projects above the right hilum.

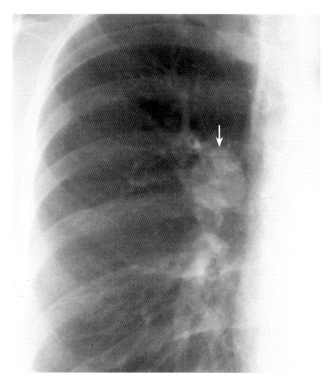

Fig. 8.**9 Bronchial adenoma.** A well circumscribed, round lesion (arrow) projects into the upper pole of the right hilum.

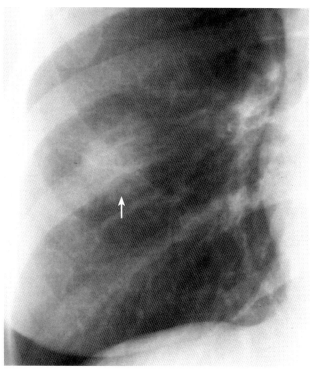

Fig. 8.**10 Bronchial adenoma.** A solitary, slightly lobulated lesion (arrow) is seen in the right middle lobe.

### Table 8.1 (Cont.) Pulmonary Nodules and Mass Lesions

| Disease | Radiographic Findings | Comments |
|---|---|---|
| **Hamartoma (Fig. 8.11 and 29.12)** | Solitary, well-circumscribed, and often lobulated lesion in the lung periphery measuring up to 4 cm in diameter. Calcifications occur in less than 10 % of cases and are virtually diagnostic when they resemble popcorn (multiple punctate calcifications throughout the lesion). Rarely, radiolucent areas (fat) can be seen within the lesion. | Peak incidence in the sixth decade (similar to bronchogenic carcinoma) with only 6 % occurring in patients under 30. *"Multiple pulmonary fibroleiomyomatous hamartomas"* can be considered a related condition that is extremely rare. |
| **Papilloma** | Solitary, or more commonly multiple, well-defined nodules that frequently cavitate. When they are centrally located in the bronchial lumen, they may present as segmental atelectatis and obstructive pneumonitis. | Most common laryngeal tumor in children, but rare in adults. Bronchopulmonary papillomas develop only rarely in the absence of laryngeal or tracheal lesions. |
| **Mesenchymal tumors (e.g., leiomyoma, lipoma, hemangioma, teratoma, chemodectoma, and neurogenic tumors)** | Rare, usually solitary, and well-defined lesions. | Except for hemoptysis in hemangiomas, these lesions are in the majority of cases asymptomatic. Malignant counterparts of these mesenchymal tumors may very rarely also originate in the lung, but represent usually hematogenous metastases from a sarcoma located in another organ. |
| **Bronchioloalveolar carcinoma (alveolar cell carcinoma) (Fig. 8.13)** | Local form (75 %). Well-circumscribed focal mass in peripheral/subpleural location, often associated with linear strands ("rabbit ears" or "tail sign") extending from the lesion to the pleura (desmoplastic reaction). Larger lesions (> 4 cm) may become ill-defined with spiculated margins ("sunburst" appearance). Tumor may surround aerated bronchus ("open bronchus sign"). The earliest stage may present with ground-glass haziness and bubble-like hyperlucencies (pseudocavitation) caused by dilatation of intact airspace from desmoplastic reaction. Diffuse form (25 %) presents as airspace consolidation with air bronchograms and poorly marginated borders or multiple bilateral poorly or well-defined nodules. Pleural effusions are associated in 10 % of cases. | Considered to be a variant of bronchogenic adenocarcinoma with mucinous (80 %) and nonmucinous (20 %) subtypes. Occurs in patients between 40 and 70 years of age without sex predilection. May be asymptomatic or presenting with cough (50 %), shortness of breath (15 %), weight loss (12 %), hemoptysis (10 %) and/or fever (8 %). Risk factors include smoking, pulmonary fibrosis (e.g. scleroderma) and localized scarring (e.g. secondary to tuberculosis or infarction). Localized form tends to be slowly progressive with 70 % surgical cure rate of tumors < 3 cm. Tumor spread occurs most frequently by tracheobronchial dissemination of detached cells to the ipsilateral or contralateral lung. |

*(continues on page 164)*

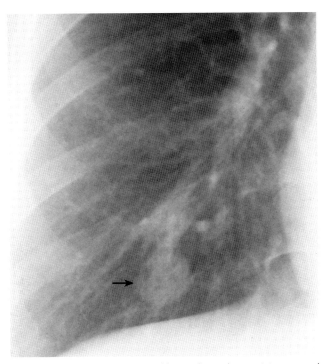

Fig. 8.**11** **Hamartoma.** A round lesion (arrow) containing several small radiolucent foci (fat) is seen in the right lower lobe.

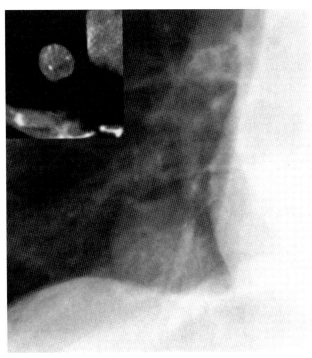

Fig. 8.**12** **Hamartoma.** A solitary nodule in the right lower lobe projects into the right cardiophrenic angle. Insert: popcorn calcifications are seen within the lesion with computed tomography.

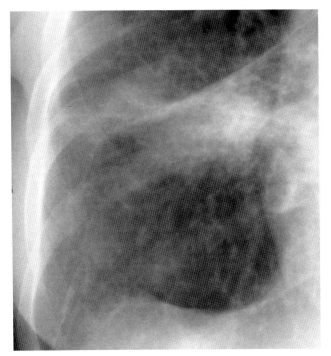

Fig. 8.**13** **Bronchioloalveolar carcinoma.** A poorly-defined mass with a few linear strands extending from the lesion toward the pleura is seen in the right middle lobe. Reticulonodular densities in the lower-lung field suggest spreading of the disease beyond the primary lesion.

**Table 8.1 (Cont.) Pulmonary Nodules and Mass Lesions**

| Disease | Radiographic Findings | Comments |
|---|---|---|
| **Bronchogenic carcinoma (Figs. 8.14, 8.15 and 8.16)** | Relatively poorly-defined nodule or mass with slight upper lobe predilection is a common presentation. Adenocarcinomas and large cell carcinomas tend to be located in the lung periphery, whereas squamous cell carcinomas and small cell carcinomas are typically located centrally. Central lesions commonly present with segmental or lobar atelectasis and obstructive pneumonitis. The "Golden S sign" is found when a central convex tumor bulge on the interlobar fissure is associated with atelectasis producing a concave deformity of the distal interlobar fissure. Cavitation occurs in 20% of squamous cell carcinomas and 6% of large cell carcinomas. The presence of one or a few eccentric tumor calcifications is rare and may be caused by either a tumor engulfing a calcified granuloma, dystrophic calcifications in tumor necrosis, or calcified mucus in adenocarcinomas. The demonstration of diffuse, laminated or central calcifications virtually rules out a bronchogenic carcinoma. Air bronchograms are typically also absent except in bronchioloalveolar carcinomas that are dealt with separately in this table. Ipsilateral hilar and mediastinal tumor involvement is common and may even be the only initial presentation of small cell carcinomas. Pleural effusions (15%) and chest wall involvement (10%) including erosions in the adjacent ribs and spine may also be evident. Distant bony metastases tend to be predominantly osteolytic, but occasionally are osteoblastic in adenocarcinomas and small cell carcinomas. | Most common cause of cancer-related death in men and women. Histologically 4 types are differentiated: 1. Adenocarcinomas (50%); 2. Squamous cell carcinomas (30%); 3. Undifferentiated small cell carcinomas (15%); 4. Undifferentiated large cell carcinomas (5%). Clinically son-small cell carcinomas are frequently differentiated from small cell carcinomas. Presents in patients ranging in age from 40 to 80 years (mean 55 to 60 years) with a male/female ratio of 1.5:1. May be asymptomatic (especially with peripheral tumors) or present with cough (75%), hemoptysis (50%), pneumonitis (40%) and/or pleurisy (10%). Initial symptoms may also be related to distant metastases (e.g. CNS, bone, liver, or adrenals) or paraneoplastic syndromes. Approximately 85% of all tumors are attributable to cigarette smoking. Other risk factors include exposure to second hand smoke, radon gas, asbestos, and arsenic, previous radiotherapy, pulmonary fibrosis and scars related to infarcts and tuberculosis. *Pancoast (superior sulcus) tumors (5%)* arise in the apex of the lung, present as unilateral apical mass or pleural cap that is commonly associated with soft tissue invasion and bone destruction. Symptoms include pain and weakness of the ipsilateral shoulder and arm, swelling of the arm and Horner syndrome (exopthalmos, ptosis, myosis, and anhidrosis). |
| **Metastases (Fig. 8.17)** | Solitary or multiple, usually well-circumscribed lesions ranging from a few millimeters to several centimeters in diameter with some lower lobe predilection. Cavitation occurs in 4%, whereas calcification is virtually limited to metastases from osteosarcomas, other bone-forming sarcomas, and mucinous adenocarcinomas. | Hematogenous metastases are multiple in 75%. Contrary to the lymphatic tumor spread in the lung, hematogeneous metastases seldom cause clinical symptoms. Metastases with an unknown primary tumor commonly originate from breast, kidney, or thyroid carcinomas. Nodules from *Kaposi's sarcoma* in AIDS patients are usually poorly defined (Fig. 8.**18**). |

*(continues on page 166)*

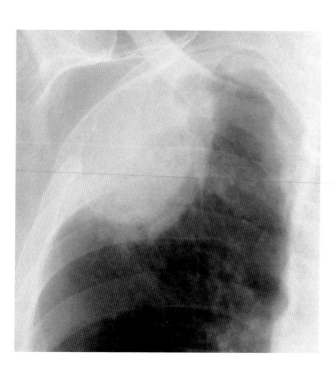

Fig. 8.**14 Bronchogenic carcinoma.** A large peripheral mass with invasion of the adjacent chest wall and partial destruction of the right third and fourth rib is seen.

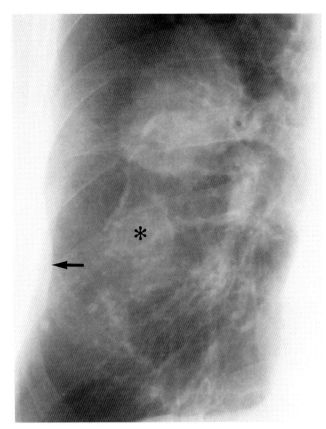

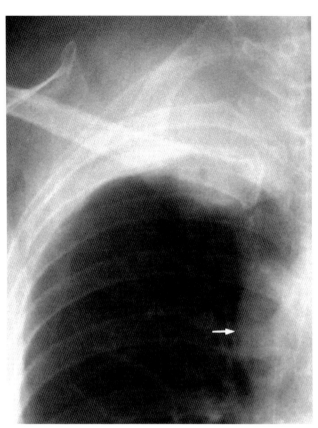

Fig. 8.**15** **Bronchogenic carcinoma.** A large bronchogenic carcinoma has developed adjacent to the right hilum in this patient with asbestosis evident from interstitial thickening in the paracardiac area, emphysematous changes, pleural plaques (arrow) and posterior pleural calcifications seen face on (asterisk).

Fig. 8.**16** **Bronchogenic carcinoma** (Pancoast tumor). A right apical mass with destruction of the right second rib posteriorly and right paratracheal lymph node metastases (arrow) is seen.

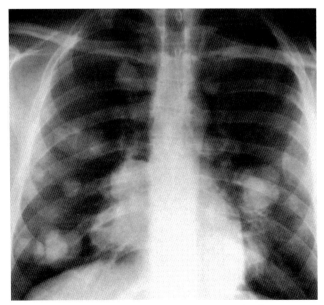

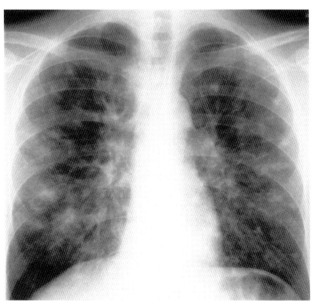

Fig. 8.**17** **Hematogenous metastases** from renal cell carcinoma. Multiple, well-circumscribed nodules of different sizes with slight lower lobe predilection are seen bilaterally.

Fig. 8.**18** **Kaposi's sarcoma.** Multiple poorly defined nodular opacities are scattered throughout both lungs of this male homosexual with AIDS.

## Table 8.1 (Cont.) Pulmonary Nodules and Mass Lesions

| Disease | Radiographic Findings | Comments |
|---|---|---|
| Lymphoma (Fig. 8.19) | Single or, more commonly, multiple nodular lesions with well-circumscribed or shaggy borders. Air bronchograms can often be found, since bronchial obstruction is very rare. In the majority of cases hilar and/or mediastinal lymphoma manifestations are associated. Cavitation is rare. | A manifestation of primary and secondary non-Hodgkin's lymphoma. Secondary Hodgkin's disease presents more commonly as a large mass than as multiple pulmonary nodules. |
| Multiple myeloma (plasmacytoma) | Solitary or multiple pulmonary masses of varying sizes. | An extrapleural mass originating from a destructive rib lesion and protruding into the lung parenchyma is a more common manifestation. |
| Amyloidosis (nodular form) | Single or, more often, multiple nodules up to several centimeters in diameter. Cavitation and calcification occur. | This nodular, parenchymal form seldom causes clinical symptoms and has a better prognosis than both the tracheobronchial (obstructive) and diffuse interstitial forms. |
| Abscess and septic emboli (Figs. 8.20 and 8.21) | Solitary or multiple round lesions ranging from 1 cm to several cm in diameter. Predilection for lower lobes and posterior segments of upper lobes. Cavitation is very common. An airborne abscess often presents originally as a poorly-defined lesion that becomes progressively better demarcated with time, whereas septic emboli present initially as well-circumscribed lesions that become more fuzzy with healing. | Staphylococcus is the most common organism. A single abscess is usually present with inhalation or aspiration of the organism, whereas multiple abscesses suggest pyemia with septic emboli. Common sources for the latter are endocarditis and septic thrombophlebitis (e.g., in drug abusers, patients with indwelling catheters or arteriovenous shunts for hemodialysis, and with pharyngeal or pelvic infections) . |
| Tuberculoma | Usually solitary and well-circumscribed lesion ranging usually from 0.5 to 4 cm in diameter. Calcifications and "satellite" lesions (small densities in immediate vicinity) are found frequently. Cavitation is extremely uncommon. Hilar lymph node calcification and scarring are often present. | Tuberculomas are late manifestations of either primary or postprimary tuberculosis. Predilection for upper lobes and posterior segments. In *atypical mycobacterial infection* multiple bilateral small nodules measuring less than 1 cm are common, but occasionally much lager nodules are encountered (Fig. 8.**22**). |
| Histoplasmoma (Fig. 8.23) | One or several well-circumscribed, round lesion(s) up to 3 cm in diameter. Predilection for lower lobes, Calcification common and often in the center ("target" appearance). "Satellite" lesions may be present. Cavitation is rare. | Hilar lymph node calcifications are commonly associated. |

*(continues on page 168)*

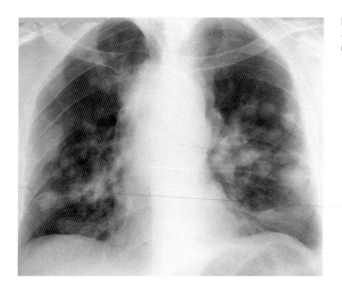

Fig. 8.**19** **Non-Hodgkin's lymphoma.** Multiple, relatively poorly-defined nodules are seen bilaterally. Note also the hilar and, particularly, mediastinal lymphadenopathy.

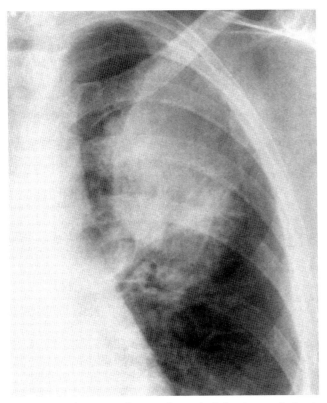

Fig. 8.**20 Pulmonary abscess.** A poorly-defined mass lesion is seen in the left upper lobe.

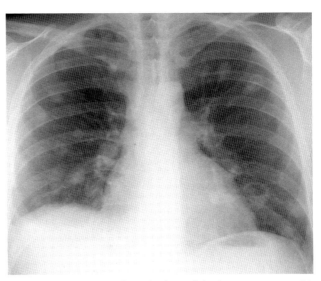

Fig. 8.**21 Septic emboll.** Multiple nodular lesions are seen bi-laterally, some of which have cavitated and contain air-fluid levels.

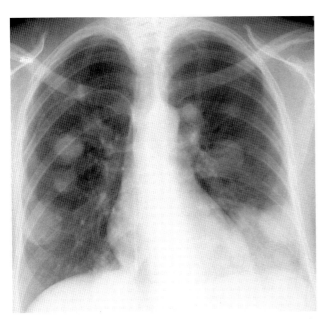

Fig. 8.**22 Atypical mycobacterial infection in AIDS.** Multiple, bi-lateral, well circumscribed, large nodules of varying sizes are seen. This is an unusual presentation of the disease.

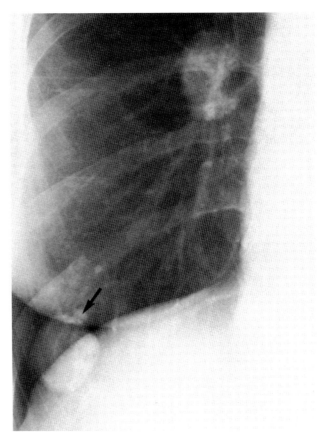

Fig. 8.**23 Histoplasmomas.** Two well-circumscribed lesions, one projecting into the right hilum and the other into the right costophrenic angle, are seen. Note also the small satellite lesion (arrow) at the periphery of the right lower lobe lesion.

### Table 8.1 (Cont.) Pulmonary Nodules and Mass Lesions

| Disease | Radiographic Findings | Comments |
|---|---|---|
| **Coccidioidomycosis** (Fig. 8.24) | Solitary or multiple, well-circumscribed nodules up to 3 cm in diameter. Upper lobe predilection. Cavitation is relatively common, calcifications rather rare. | Even patients with cavitary disease are often asymptomatic. |
| **Actinomycosis Nocardiosis Blastomycosis Cryptococcosis** (Figs. 8.25 and 8.26) | Usually single, large mass lesion measuring up to 10 cm in diameter. Except for blastomycosis, cavitation is relatively common and the lower lobes are preferentially involved. Disease may extend through the pleura into the chest wall and involve the ribs. | In cryptococcosis, the lesion is characteristically pleural-based, but an effusion is uncommon. Empyema is a common complication of actinomycosis and nocardiosis only. |
| **Echinococcal disease** (Fig. 8.27) | Usually solitary, sharply circumscribed, spherical or oval mass preferentially in a lower lobe (slightly more common on the right), and ranging up to 10 cm in diameter. Large lesions may have bizarre, polycystic, lobulated outlines. Calcification virtually never occurs in lung lesions. | Cyst wall is composed of 3 layers: pericystic (fibrous reaction formed by host), exocystic (chitinous outer cyst membrane), and endocystic (thin inner lining of syncytial cells). Air entering between the pericystic and exocystic layers produces a crescent-shaped, peripheral radiolucency: the "double arch" sign, found in 5%. After rupturing into a bronchus, an air-fluid level is found with the endocyst floating on the surface, producing the "water lily" sign or "camelot sign." |
| **Hypersensitivity aspergillosis with mucoid impaction** (Fig. 8.28) | Solitary or, less common, multiple, round, oval or elliptical opacities caused by plugs in dilated, usually second-order bronchi. Upper lobes are preferentially involved. Opacifications may also have a "Y" or "V" configuration when a bronchial bifurcation is plugged. | Hypersensitivity aspergillosis is usually associated with asthma or pre-existing chronic bronchial disease. Other forms of secondary aspergillosis include aspergillomas in cavitary lesions and single or multiple, occasionally cavitary consolidations in patients with chronic debilitating diseases. Primary aspergillosis is exceedingly rare and presents as homogeneous consolidation that may progress to abscess formation. *Bronchocentric granulomatosis (Liebow)* may be considered a variant of hypersensitivity aspergillosis and appears both clinically and radiographically in a similar fashion (Fig. 8.**29**). |

*(continues on page 170)*

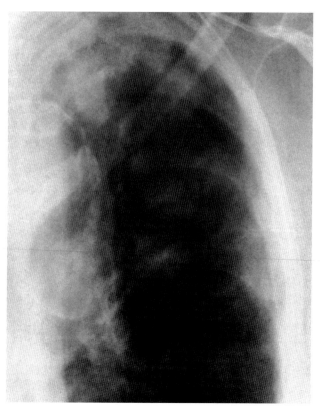

Fig. 8.**24 Coccidioidomycosis.** Several nodular lesions are seen in the left upper lobe in this patient with preexisting, unrelated chronic pulmonary and pleural changes.

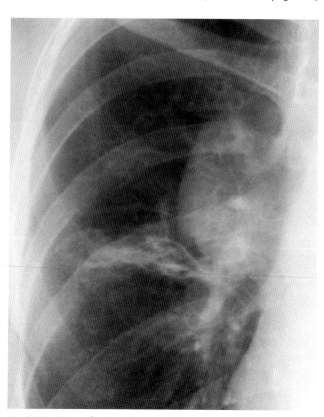

Fig. 8.**25 Nocardiosis.** A large ovoid mass projects into the upper pole of the right hilum in this patient with AIDS. Interstitial infiltrates caused by atypical mycobacterial infection are also evident.

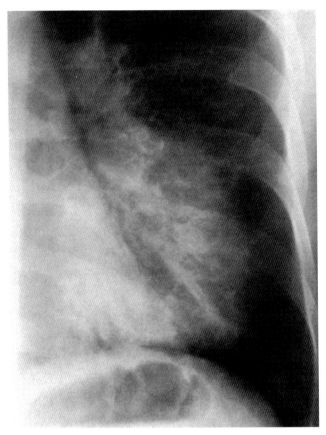

Fig. 8.**26** **Cryptococcosis.** A large, well-defined mass is seen in the left lower lobe in this patient with AIDS. There is also mild left hilar adenopathy, which is unusual for this disease.

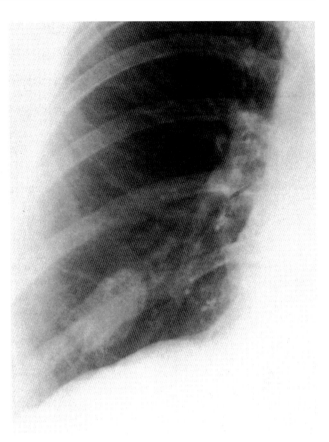

Fig. 8.**27** **Echinococcus.** A solitary, oval-shaped and slightly lobulated lesion is seen in the right lower lobe.

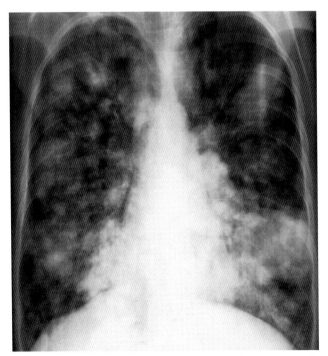

Fig. 8.**28** **Hypersensitivity aspergillosis** complicating cystic fibrosis. Multiple round opacities and areas of consolidations are seen throughout both lungs. This is an unusually extensive involvement by hypersensitivity aspergillosis. More often the disease presents as solitary lesion.

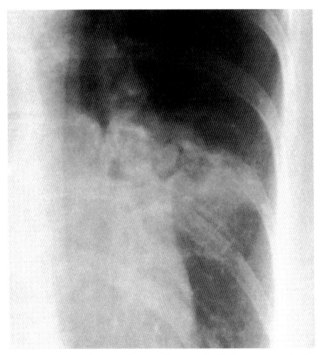

Fig. 8.**29** **Bronchocentric granulomatosis Liebow.** A poorly defined mass lesion silhouetting the left cardiac border is seen in the lingula.

## Table 8.1 (Cont.) Pulmonary Nodules and Mass Lesions

| Disease | Radiographic Findings | Comments |
|---|---|---|
| **Congenital bronchial atresia** | Well-circumscribed, somewhat elliptical mass, caused by mucus accumulated in a bronchus peripheral to the point of stenosis or atresia. Usually located in an upper lobe, most commonly in the apicoposterior segment of the left side. | This anomaly rarely causes symptoms and usually is discovered in a screening chest radiograph in children or young adults. |
| **Inflammatory pseudo-tumor (Fig. 8.30)** | Solitary nodule or homogeneous area of consolidation, ranging up to 7 cm in diameter and often mimicking a primary carcinoma. | May represent the sequela of an unresolved pneumonia, although a history of acute respiratory illness is not always available. An inflammatory pseudotumor should not be confused with a so-called "pseudotumor" of a pleural fissure resulting from loculated fluid accumulation. |
| **Pseudolymphoma** | Nodular lesions less common than parenchymal consolidations that characteristically contain air bronchograms. In contrast to pulmonary lymphoma, hilar and mediastinal lymph nodes are never involved. | May represent a modified form of an inflammatory pseudotumor. |
| **Lipoid pneumonia (Fig. 8.31)** | Peripheral, usually well-defined mass measuring up to several centimeters in diameter and preferentially being located in the posterior segments. Occasionally, a shaggy outline is found caused by linear shadows (thickened interlobular septa) radiating from the periphery of the lesion. | Caused by chronic aspiration of vegetable, animal, or mineral oils. May mimic peripheral bronchogenic carcinoma. |
| **Pulmonary infarct (Fig. 8.32)** | Solitary or multiple homogeneous consolidations abutting the pleural surface. Nodular densities are less common. A "Hampton's hump" (pleural-based semicircular consolidation) is characteristic but rare. Resolution occurs through a gradual decrease in size ("melting ice cube sign"). | Other signs of pulmonary thromboembolism are often associated, and include: 1 loss of lung volume with elevation of the ipsilateral diaphragm, 2 oligemia resulting in increasing radiolucency of affected lung areas (Westermark sign), 3 pleural effusions, 4 enlargement of the hilar pulmonary artery and azygos vein and 5 acute cardiac enlargement (cor pulmonale). |
| **Pulmonary hematoma (Fig. 8.33)** | Single or multiple, well-circumscribed, round or oval lesions, usually measuring between 2 and 6 cm. Peripheral subpleural location immediately underlying the point of maximum impact is characteristic. Air-fluid level may be present. Lesion may initially be masked by surrounding lung contusion. | Results from bleeding into a parenchymal laceration or a traumatic cyst. Gradual decrease in size over several weeks or months. |

*(continues on page 172)*

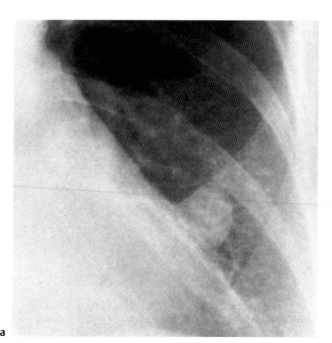
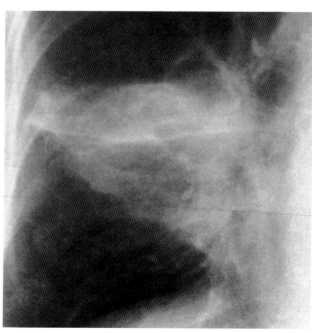

a b

Fig. 8.**30 a, b** **Inflammatory pseudotumors** (2 cases). A solitary nodule in the left lower lobe is seen in **a** and a larger mass lesion involving the right middle lobe is present in **b**. Both cases underwent surgery, since a bronchogenic carcinoma was suspected.

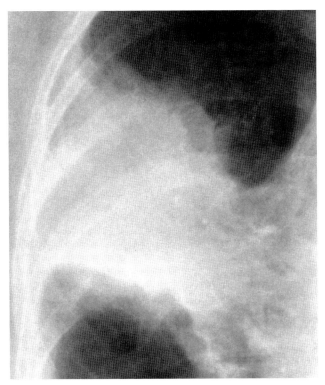

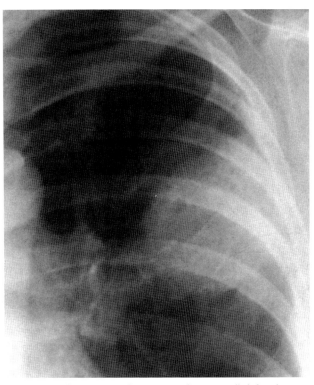

Fig. 8.**31**   **Lipoid pneumonia.** A peripheral mass with somewhat shaggy outline is seen.

Fig. 8.**32**   **Pulmonary infarct.** A solitary, well-defined mass ("Hampton's hump") abutting the diaphragmatic pleura is seen.

Fig. 8.**33**   **Pulmonary hematoma.** A mass lesion in the right upper lobe is seen in this patient after he was shot.

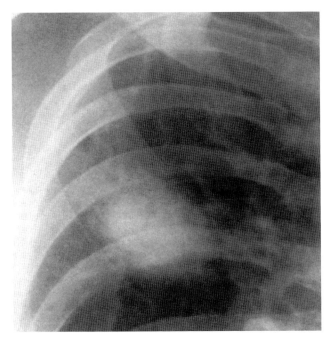

## Table 8.1 (Cont.) Pulmonary Nodules and Mass Lesions

| Disease | Radiographic Findings | Comments |
|---|---|---|
| **Progressive massive fibrosis (PMF)** (Fig. 8.34) | Large, often bilateral, but usually asymmetric, spindle-shaped, mass lesions in the upper half of the lungs. The lateral border paralleling the rib cage is usually better defined than the medial border. May contain calcifications and cavitate (due to either ischemic necrosis or superimposed tuberculosis). Tend to migrate toward the hila over the years. | PMF is associated with *pneumoconiosis* (especially coal miner's lung and silicosis) although radiographic evidence of the underlying pneumoconiosis may occasionally not be obvious. Similar conglomerate masses of fibrosis may occasionally be found with sarcoidosis where they may contain air bronchograms. |
| **Sarcoidosis** (Fig. 8.35) | Multiple, well-circumscribed nodules measuring up to 2 cm and conglomerate masses of fibrosis. Commonly associated with reticulonodular interstitial disease or fibrosis (honeycombing). Hilar and mediastinal lymphadenopathy may also be present. | This is a relatively rare manifestation of sarcoidosis. |
| **Wegener's granulomatosis** (Fig. 8.36) | Solitary or, more often, multiple, fairly well-circumscribed nodules ranging from less than 1 cm to 10 cm in diameter. Cavitation is common. Alveolar infiltrates may be associated. Pleural effusion is not unusual. Hilar lymph node enlargement is very rare. | Multiple nodules simulating metastases are the most common pulmonary presentation of Wegener's granulomatosis. In the limited form, lungs are the only affected organ, whereas in the full-blown form of Wegener's granulomatosis, kidneys, nose, and paranasal sinuses are involved also. The radiologic manifestations of the *lymphomatoid variant of Wegener's granulomatosis* in the lung are virtually identical to those of Wegener's granulomatosis, but the paranasal sinuses are characteristically not involved with the former. |
| **Polyarteritis nodosa** (Fig. 8.37) | Poorly-defined nodules with patchy consolidations. The fleeting nature of pulmonary manifestations is characteristic. | Renal and gastrointestinal symptoms usually predominant. Poor prognosis. Some cases have histories of drug reactions: *"hypersensitivity angiitis."* *Churg-Strauss syndrome* is a variant of polyarteritis nodosa presenting with allergic asthma, eosinophilia and systemic small vessel vasculitis with granulomatous inflammation. |
| **Rheumatoid necrobiotic nodules** (Fig. 8.38) | Solitary or, more commonly, multiple, well-circumscribed peripheral nodules measuring a few millimeters to several centimeters. Lower lobe predilection. Cavitation common. | Necrobiotic nodules are a rare manifestation of rheumatoid lung disease. Nodules may wax and wane in concert with subcutaneous nodules. *Caplan's syndrome:* necrobiotic nodules and rheumatoid arthritis in pneumoconicosis. Calcifications can occur in these nodules. |

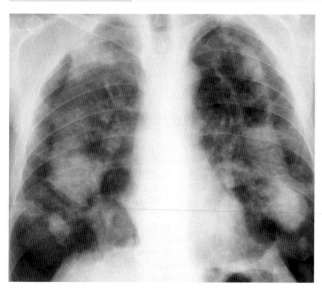

Fig. 8.**34 Progressive massive fibrosis** (PMF) in coal miner's lung. Besides smaller areas of fibrosis, one larger, spindle-shaped opacity is seen in each lung, extending from the mid-lung fields into the upper lobes. The lateral borders of these opacities characteristically are better defined than are the medial borders, Note also that cavitation in the upper half of the left mass has occurred, probably due to ischemic necrosis, but superimposed tuberculosis cannot be ruled out radiographically.

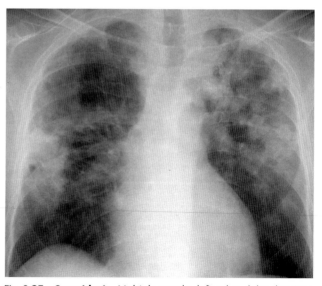

Fig. 8.**35 Sarcoidosis.** Multiple poorly defined nodular densities are seen bilaterally in the mid and upper lung zones associated with interstitial lung disease including honeycombing and mild hilar lymphadenopathy. Beginning formation of conglomerate fibrotic masses in the lung periphery is caused by the coalescence of the nodular lesions.

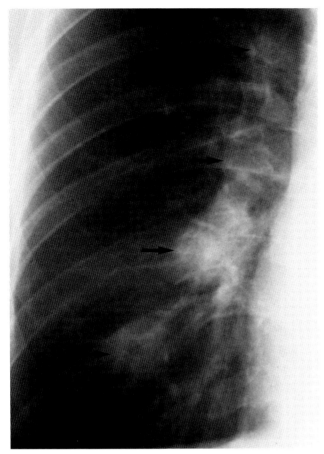

Fig. 8.**36 Wegener's granulomatosis.** Four fairly well-circumscribed nodules (arrows) are seen in the right lung. Incipient central cavitation is recognizable in the lowest nodule.

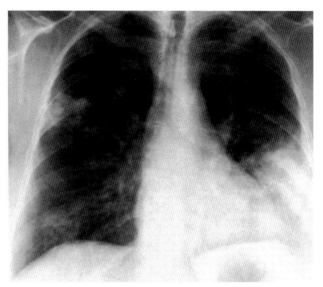

Fig. 8.**37 Polyarteritis nodosa.** Poorly defined nodules with patchy consolidations are seen involving both lungs.

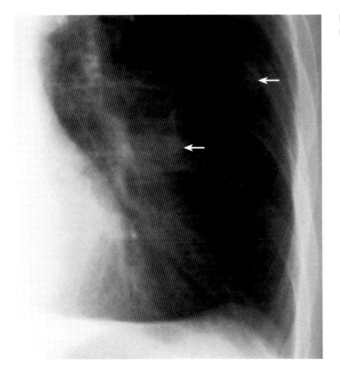

Fig. 8.**38 Rheumatoid necrobiotic** nodules. Two nodules (arrows) are associated with slightly increased interstitial markings.

# 9 Pulmonary Cavitary and Cystic Lesions

Pulmonary cavitary and cystic lesions are characterized by their central air content. Cavities usually result from central necrosis within a lesion and the subsequent expulsion of the necrotic material into the bronchial system. Rupture of a fluid-filled cyst or infection of a bulla may produce a similar radiographic appearance. Cavities often contain fluid that appears as an air-fluid level on radiographs performed with horizontal beam. Air-fluid levels occur when a lesion with a liquid content ruptures into the tracheobronchial system and part of its content is expelled, or when both gas and pus are produced by bacteria. A cavitary lesion with an air-fluid level is, however, not pathognomonic of a pulmonary lesion (e.g., a lung abscess), but also can be encountered in the event of a *loculated hydropneumothorax* (e.g., loculated empyema secondary to the bronchopleural fistula). Radiologic differentiation of these two entities is, however, made possible by the fact that a pulmonary cavity tends to be spherical and, consequently, the length of the air-fluid level is very similar on frontal, lateral, and decubitus films. A loculated hydropneumothorax, however, is virtually never spherical, since it must conform in shape to the adjacent chest wall and, consequently, the length of the air-fluid level varies widely between different projections (Fig. 9.1).

Cystic lesions can be mimicked by plastic (radiolucent) spheres inserted in the past into the extrapleural space to collapse the adjacent lung for the treatment of tuberculosis. Since these spheres were often not water-tight, small amounts of fluid could collect in them, mimicking small air-fluid levels on upright films. Nowadays, cystic lesions with or without air-fluid levels can be simulated by both *hiatal* and *diaphragmatic hernias* (congenital or posttraumatic), when they contain the stomach or loops of bowel. Characteristic of these hernias is, however, a considerable change in the size and shape of the lesions between subsequent radiographs.

Cavitary lesions can be differentiated from each other by their size, location, wall thickness, number and by the nature of both their inner lining (smooth or irregular) and content (fluid versus mass).

The cavity wall thickness can be described as hairline (1 mm or less), thin (2 to 4 mm) and thick (5 mm and more) (Fig. 9.2). Hairline cavities are invariably associated with benign conditions such as bullae, blebs and pneumatoceles. The vast majority of thin-walled cavities are also found with a variety of benign lesions including chronic infections such as coccidiodomycosis, whereas thick-walled cavities are equally divided between benign and malignant conditions such as lung abscess, primary and metastatic carcinoma, and Wegener's granulomatosis. However an extremely thick cavity wall exceeding 15 mm is highly suspicious of a malignant neoplasm.

A solitary cavitary lung lesion is frequently found in a pulmonary abscess, a malignant neoplasm or a lung cyst (congenital or posttraumatic). Multiple cavitary lung lesions suggest Wegener's granulomatosis and septic emboli or metastatic disease. The inner lining of a cavity is usually nodular in a bronchogenic carcinoma, shaggy in an acute lung abscess and smooth in most other lesions.

Fluid in the presence of gas can be diagnosed in a cavitary lesion by the demonstration of an air-fluid level on radiographs taken with horizontal beam. The intracavitary fluid

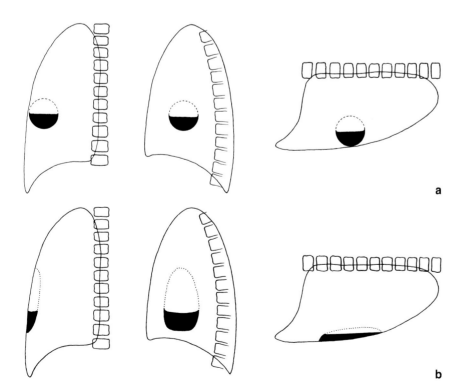

Fig. 9.**1 a, b Differentiation between air-fluid levels**, **a** in a peripheral pulmonary cavity and **b** in a loculated hydropneumothorax. **a** A pulmonary cavity tends to be spherical and therefore an air-fluid level in such a lesion has the same length in anteroposterior, lateral, and decubitus films. **b** A loculated hydropneumothorax must conform to the chest wall and is therefore never spherical. The length of the air-fluid level varies considerably between different projections as shown here in the anteroposterior, lateral, and decubitus films.

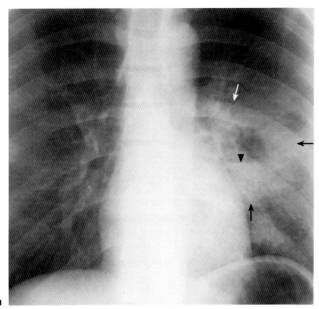

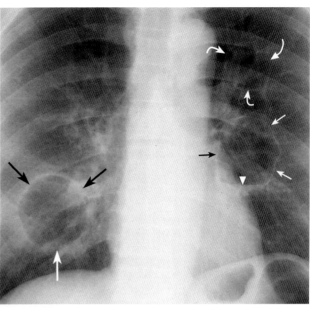

a

b

Fig. 9.**2   Cavitary lesions with variable wall thickness. a** A lung abscess (arrows) presenting as poorly defined thick-walled cavitary lesion with air-fluid (pus) level (arrowhead) is seen in the left lower lobe. **b** Four years later a pneumatocele with hairline wall (small ar- rows) and tiny fluid level (arrowhead) has replaced the abscess. A second pneumatocele (curved arrows) is seen more cephalad. A thin-walled cyst (large arrows) representing another healing ab- scess is now seen in the right lower lobe.

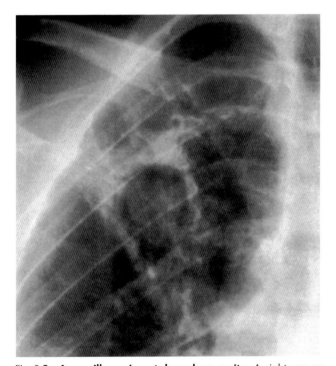

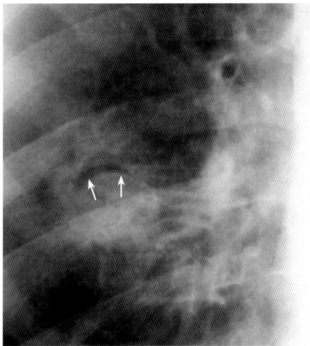

Fig. 9.**3   Aspergilloma in a tuberculous cavity.** A right upper lobe cavity is seen containing a mass lesion. Note also the pericavi- tary infiltrates indicating still-active tuberculosis.

Fig. 9.**4   Aspergilloma in old abscess cavity.** The aspergilloma is separated from the wall of the cavity by a crescent-shaped air space (arrows).

may be serous or sanguinous or represent pus or liquefied necrotic tissue. Besides fluid, a mass can also be found within a cavitary lesion. With regard to the size of the cavity, the mass can be quite small or occupy most of the cavitary space. In the latter case, the mass is only separated from the wall of the cavity by a crescent-shaped air space. Most commonly, intracavitary mass lesions represent *mycetomas*, especially *aspergillomas* (Figs. 9.**3** and 9.**4**). They can be found in infec- tious (particularly tuberculous), tumoral, bronchiectatic, and cystic cavities that do not contain any fluid. Similar intracavi- tary masses can be produced by necrotic tumor fragments in carcinomas, sequestered necrotic lung tissue in klebsiella or, rarely, in pneumococcal pneumonias, a blood clot, or by the collapsed membrane of a ruptured echinococcal cyst floating on top of the fluid ("water-lily" or "camelot" sign).

The differential diagnosis of various cavitary and cystic le- sions measuring 1 cm or more in diameter is given in Table 9.**1**.

## Table 9.1    Solitary or Multiple Cavitary and Cystic Pulmonary Lesions

| Disease | Radiographic Findings | Comments |
|---|---|---|
| **Bronchogenic cyst (congenital or traumatic)** | Solitary thin-walled lesion with or without air-fluid level. | Congenital cysts are characteristically located in medial third of the lungs with lower lobe predilection. |
| **Intralobar bronchopulmonary sequestration (Fig. 9.5)** | Solitary, unilocular, or multilocular cystic mass that may or may not contain air-fluid levels. Cyst walls are thick or thin. | Lesion is usually contiguous with the diaphragm and characteristically located in a posterobasal segment of a lower lobe (left to right ratio 3 : 1). Masking of lesion by surrounding pneumonia is possible. |
| **Congenital cystic adenomatoid malformation (Fig. 9.6 and 9.7)** | Multilocular cystic mass with or without air-fluid levels, similar to bronchopulmonary sequestration, but involves at least an entire lobe without predilection. The volume of the affected lung is usually increased or, less commonly, decreased. Three types are differentiated. Type I: Single or multiple large cysts exceeding 20 mm in diameter. DD: *Congenital lobar emphysema* involving LUL (40 %), RML (35 %), RUL (20 %), or two lobes (5 %). Type II: Multiple cysts measuring 5 to 12 mm in diameter. Type III: Solitary large bulky mass with 3 to 5 mm small microcysts. | Involves characteristically one lobe, but occasionally two lobes or both lungs are affected. Usually diagnosed in infancy, but may occasionally be diagnosed first in older children or adolescents. May be part of a wider spectrum that includes also bronchogenic cysts and sequestrations. DD: *Diaphragmetic hernia* containing bowel loops (Fig. 9.**8**) and extensive cystic bronchiectases (Fig. 9.**9**). |

*(continues on page 178)*

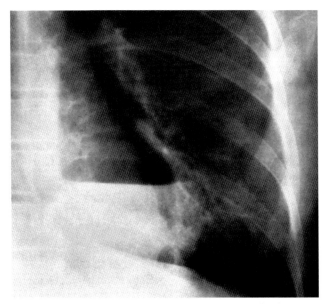

Fig. 9.**5**  **Intralobar sequestration.** A cystic mass with a large air-fluid level is seen in the posterobasal segment of the left lower lobe.

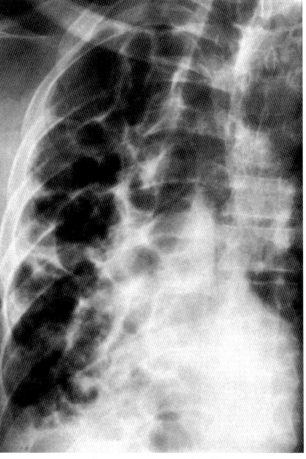

Fig. 9.**6**  **Congenital cystic adenomatoid malformation (type I).** A multilocular cystic mass has replaced the right lung. Note also the significant loss of volume that helps to differentiate this condition from a large diaphragmatic hernia containing bowel loops.

**Table 9.1   (Cont.) Solitary or Multiple Cavitary and Cystic Pulmonary Lesions**

| Disease | Radiographic Findings | Comments |
|---|---|---|
| Pulmonary papillomatosis | Multiple, well-defined nodules that frequently cavitate and then resemble cystic bronchiectases. | Most common laryngeal tumor in children, but rare in adults. Pulmonary papillomas seldom develop in the absence of laryngeal or tracheal lesions. |
| Bronchogenic carcinoma (Fig. 9.10) | Solitary, usually thick-walled cavity with irregular inner lining. A smooth, thin-walled cavity is a rare presentation. Necrotic tumor tissue may simulate mycetoma. Air-fluid levels are uncommon. | Cavitation occurs in up to 10% of cases of bronchogenic carcinoma, most commonly in squamous cell carcinomas, especially in the upper lobes, and undifferentiated large cell carcinomas, rarely in adenocarcinomas, and never in small cell carcinomas |
| Metastases, hematogenous (Fig. 9.11) | Multiple nodules of different sizes with thin or thick-walled cavities developing in a varying percentages of lesions (few to almost all). | Cavitation less common than in bronchogenic carcinoma. Metastases frequently originate from squamous cell carcinoma of the head and neck (thin-walled cavities), or gynecologic tumors and sarcomas (thick-walled cavities). |
| Lymphoma (Fig. 9.12) | One or more consolidations with usually thick-walled cavities that have an irregular inner lining and may contain an air-fluid level. | A manifestation of primary and secondary non-Hodgkin's lymphoma and secondary Hodgkin's disease. In secondary pulmonary involvement the disease is associated with simultaneous or past presentations in other organs (e.g., peripheral and mediastinal lymph nodes). |

*(continues on page 180)*

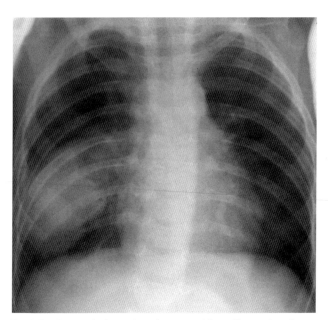

Fig. 9.**7   Congenital cystic adenomatoid malformation (type III).** A large bulky mass occupies the right middle lobe. The microcysts within the lesion cannot be appreciated.

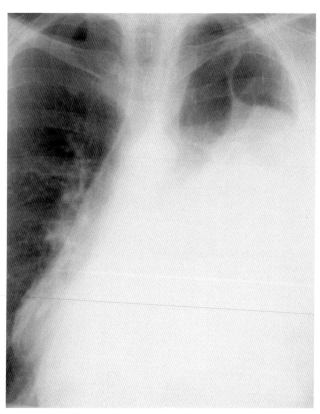

Fig. 9.**8   Diaphragmatic hernia.** The hernia occupies most of the left hemithorax with air filled bowel loops seen in its apex. Note also the shift of the heart towards the contralateral side caused by the mass effect of the hernia.

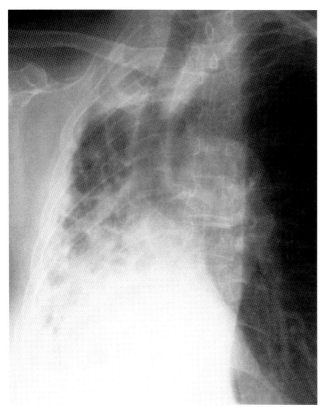

Fig. 9.**9  Cystic bronchiectasis in chronic tuberculosis.** Multiple cystic lesions with marked loss of volume are seen in the shrunken fibrotic right lung resulting in shift of heart and mediastinum towards the ipsilateral side.

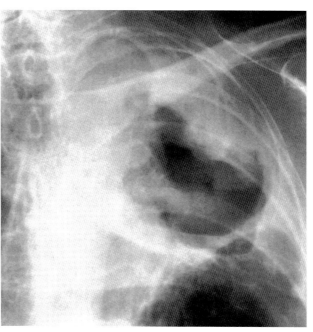

Fig. 9.**10  Bronchogenic carcinoma** (squamous cell type). A left upper lobe mass containing a large cavity with irregular nodular inner lining is seen.

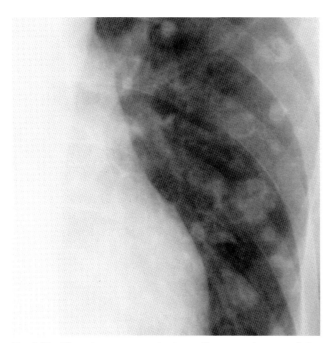

Fig. 9.**11  Hematogenous metastases from carcinoma of the hypopharynx.** Multiple, different-sized nodules are present bilaterally with a large number demonstrating central cavitation. The finding is best appreciated in the left mid and lower lung field shown here.

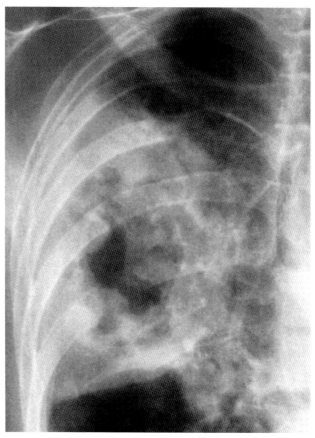

Fig. 9.**12  Non-Hodgkin's lymphoma.** A right upper lobe consolidation with irregular central cavitation is seen.

### Table 9.1    (Cont.) Solitary or Multiple Cavitary and Cystic Pulmonary Lesions

| Disease | Radiographic Findings | Comments |
|---|---|---|
| **Abscess, bacterial** | | |
| **Staphylococcus (Fig. 9.13 and 9.14)** | Single or multiple thick-walled cavities with often shaggy inner linings and air-fluid levels occur in approximately half of the patients with staphylococcus pneumonia. Pleural effusion (empyema) with or without bronchopleural fistula (pyopneumothorax) and pneumatoceles are common, particularly in children. | *Pneumatoceles* are thin-walled cystic spaces that may contain air-fluid levels, commonly found in children. Probably caused by check-valve obstruction of a communication between a peribronchial microabscess and the lumen of a bronchus. |
| **Klebsiella (Fig. 9.15)** | Single thick-walled cavity with shaggy inner border in upper lobe is characteristic. Besides an air-fluid level, one or several pieces of necrotic lung parenchyma floating like icebergs in the cavity fluid is occasionally seen indicating pulmonary gangrene. | A radiographically similar upper lobe abscess is a common finding in *Proteus pneumonias* and a rare manifestation in *pneumococcal pneumonias*. |
| **Pseudomonas Anaerobic bacteria** | Bilateral consolidations with multiple cavities predominantly in lower lobes and posterior segments characteristic. Diameter of cavities ranges from less than 1 cm to several centimeters, but majority measures less than 3 cm. Air-fluid levels are not a dominant feature and are often only conspicuous in large cavities exceeding 3 cm in diameter. Pleural effusions (empyema) are commonly associated. | Usually in patients with debilitating diseases. A Pseudomonas pneumonia is commonly acquired in the hospital. Mode of infection by inhalation (Pseudomonas) or aspiration (anaerobics) and via bloodstream. Similar radiographic findings are found in *Escherichia coli* and *Salmonella pneumonias*. |
| **Tuberculosis (Figs. 9.16 and 9.17)** | One or more thin- or thick-walled cavities with a generally smooth inner lining. High predilection for apical and posterior segment of upper lobes and superior segment of lower lobes. Air-fluid levels are rarely present. | Persistent thin-walled cavitation after chemotherapy does not necessarily indicate active disease. With *atypical mycobacterial infections* cavities (usually multiple) are even more common (Fig. 9.18). |

(continues on page 182)

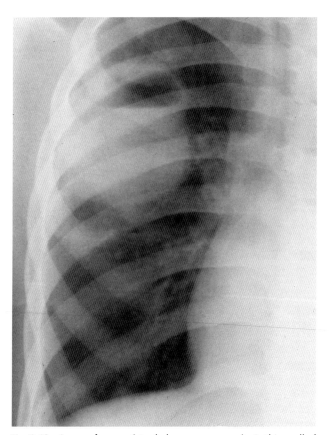

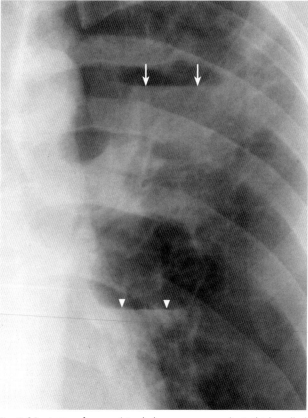

Fig. 9.**13**  **Lung abscess** (staphylococcus aureus). A thin-walled cavity with relatively smooth inner lining and air-fluid (pus) level is seen in the right upper lobe.

Fig. 9.**14**  **Lung abscess** (staphylococcus aureus). A thick-walled cavity with shaggy inner lining, air-fluid level (arrows) and surrounding infiltrate is seen in the left upper lobe. A pneumatocele with small air-fluid level (arrowheads) in the left lower lobe is the sequela of an old abscess shown in Fig. 9.**2a** 2¹/₂ years earlier.

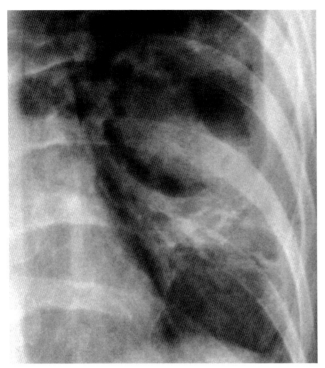

Fig. 9.**15 Klebsiella pneumonia.** A thick-walled cavity with shaggy inner border containing a large mass of necrotic lung is evident

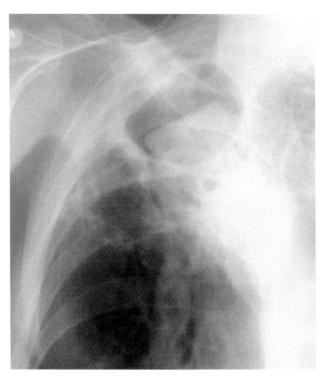

Fig. 9.**16 Tuberculous cavity with aspergilloma.** Chronic tuberculosis with a large cavity containing an aspergilloma is seen in the shrunken fibrotic and infiltrated right upper lobe surrounded by extensive apical pleural thickening.

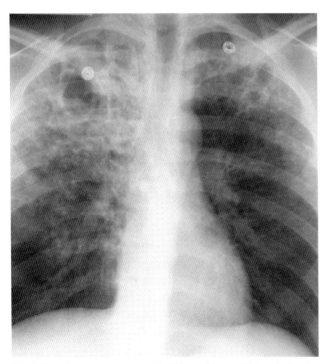

Fig. 9.**17 Cavitary tuberculosis.** Bilateral interstitial and alveolar infiltrates with several thin-walled cavities are seen in both upper lobes and the superior segments of the lower lobes.

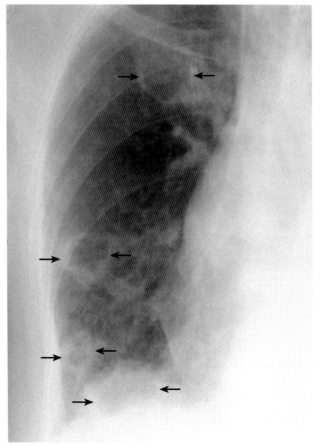

Fig. 9.**18 Atypical mycobacterial infection in AIDS.** Four irregular thin-walled cavities (arrows) are associated with reticulonodular disease.

**Table 9.1 (Cont.) Solitary or Multiple Cavitary and Cystic Pulmonary Lesions**

| Disease | Radiographic Findings | Comments |
|---|---|---|
| **Actinomycosis Nocardiosis (Fig. 9.19)** | Solitary, large, thick-walled cavitary lesion with lower lobe predilection. Extension through pleura into chest wall with rib involvement occurs. | Empyema is commonly associated with actinomycosis and nocardiosis |
| ***Fungal diseases*** | | |
| **Histoplasmosis** | One or more cavities usually located in upper lobes and indistinguishable from tuberculosis. | Tuberculosis and histoplasmosis may even coexist in the same patient. |
| **Coccidioidomycosis (Fig. 9.20** | Solitary or multiple, thin- or thick-walled, cavitary lesions. Air-fluid levels may be present. Cavitation occurs predominantly in upper lobe nodules, but, unlike tuberculosis, they are characteristically located in the anterior segments. | Very thin-walled cystic lesions, predominantly in the upper lobes, may be the sequelae of an asymptomatic or flu-like coccidioidomycosis infection. |
| **Mucormycosis (Fig. 9.21)** | Homogeneous consolidation with frequent cavitation. | Almost invariably in patient with underlying disease (e.g., diabetes, lymphoma, and leukemia). |
| **Blastomycosis Cryptococcosis (Fig. 9.22)** | Solitary mass lesion or, less commonly, multiple nodules, often with air bronchograms (> 50 %), and occasionally with cavitation (15 %) and hilar/mediastinal lymphadenopathy (20 %). | Opportunistic invaders in immunocompromised patients and diabetics. |
| **Aspergillosis Candidiasis (moniliasis)** | Cavitation occurs in patchy infiltrates. | Virtually limited to debilitated patients. Both organisms can also be found as fungus balls in cavitary lesions of various origins. |
| ***Parasitic diseases*** | | |
| **Amebiasis** | Solitary, thick-walled, right lower lobe cavity with as irregular inner surface characteristic. Right pleural effusion almost invariably present. | Pulmonary manifestation is a direct extension from a liver abscess through the diaphragm. Besides the right lower lobe, other lobes contiguous to the diaphragm and covering the liver surface can be involved occasionally. |
| **Echinococcus (Fig. 9.23)** | Solitary or less common, multiple cystic lesions with lower lobe predilection. Cystic membrane may float on top of air-fluid level ("water-lily" sign) or lie at the bottom of a dry cyst. | After rupturing into bronchus, part or, less commonly, all of the liquid content is expelled into the bronchial system. |
| **Paragonimiasis** | Usually multiple, relatively thin-walled cysts ranging from less than one to several centimeters in diameter. Local elevation or hump on inner lining characteristic. | This presentation of paragonimiasis has been limited to an endemic area in Thailand. |

*(continues on page 184)*

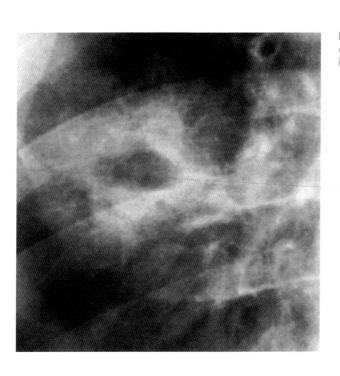

**Fig. 9.19 Actinomycosis.** A poorly-defined consolidation with central cavitation containing an air-fluid level is seen in the superior segment of the right lower lobe.

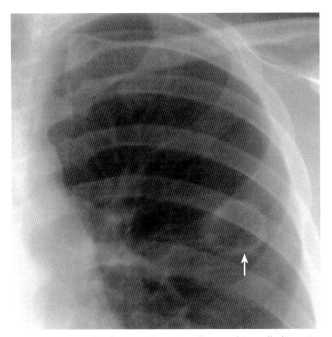

Fig. 9.**20** **Coccidioidomycosis.** A solitary thin-walled cavity (arrow) is seen in the anterior segment of the left upper lobe.

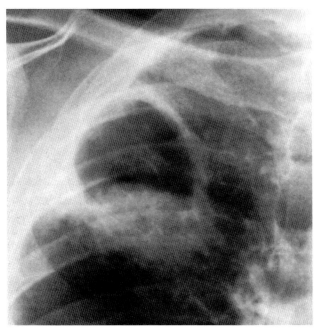

Fig. 9.**21** **Mucormycosis** in patient with diabetes. A relatively thin-walled cavity containing a mass with slightly convex upper border (mycetoma) at its base is seen in the right upper lobe.

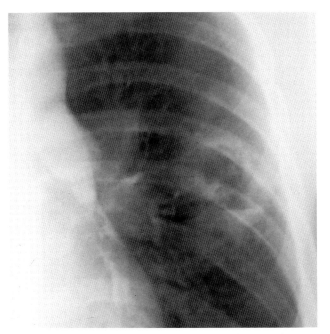

Fig. 9.**22** **Blastomycosis.** An irregular peripheral cavitary lesion is associated with left hilar and mediastinal lymphadenopathy.

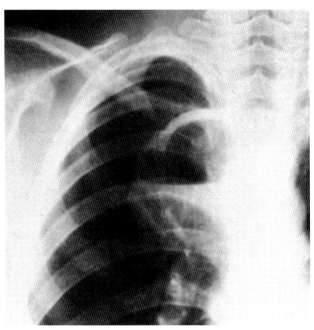

Fig. 9.**23** **Echinococcus.** A solitary cystic lesion with an air-fluid level is seen in the right upper lobe adjacent to the mediastinum.

**Table 9.1 (Cont.) Solitary or Multiple Cavitary and Cystic Pulmonary Lesions**

| Disease | Radiographic Findings | Comments |
|---|---|---|
| **Progressive massive fibrosis (PMF) in pneumoconiosis (Fig. 9.24)** | Usually thick-walled cavity with irregular inner surface in a mid and upper lung zone mass in silicosis or coal miner's lung. | Cavitation in PMF is caused more often by superimposed tuberculosis than by ischemic necrosis. |
| **Rheumatoid necrobiotic nodules** | Usually multiple, thick- or thin-walled cavitary lesions measuring a few millimeters to several centimeters with smooth inner surface and lower lobe predilection. | Both cavitary and noncavitary lesions decrease during remission and increase with exacerbation of the rheumatoid arthritis. Cavitary lesion may fill in and become homogeneous again. |
| **Wegener's granulomatosis (Fig, 9.25)** | Multiple, bilateral, thick–walled cavitary nodules with irregular inner surface characteristic. Solitary or thin-walled cystic lesions are occasionally seen. Air-fluid levels rarely occur. | Cavitation occurs in almost half of all patients. When multiple nodules are present, rarely all cavitate. |
| **Pulmonary hematoma and traumatic cyst (pneumatocele) (Fig. 9.26)** | Presents initially either as homogeneous well-circumscribed mass (hematoma) that eventually may partially evacuate into the bronchial system producing a cavitary lesion or as thin-walled cyst with or without air-fluid (blood) level measuring up to 10 cm and more in diameter. | Lesions may be seen radiographically immediately after a blunt chest trauma, but more often they are only evident hours or days later. Complete evacuation of a hematoma into the bronchial system can also produce a traumatic cyst or pneumatocele, respectively. |
| **Septic emboli (Fig. 9.27)** | Multiple, thin- or, less commonly, thick-walled, peripheral, round or wedge-shaped cavitary lesions, sometimes with air-fluid levels. | Often in patients under 40 years of age with endocarditis, septic thrombophlebitis (e.g. in intravenous drug abusers and patients with indwelling catheters or arteriovenous shunts for hemodialysis), pharyngeal and pelvic infections (e. g., septic abortion) and osteomyelitis. Cavitation in *nonseptic emboli* and *infarcts* is very rare. |
| **Bronchiectasis, cystic (Fig. 9.28)** | Multiple, relatively thin-walled cystic lesions measuring up to 3 cm in diameter, often with a tiny air-fluid level at the bottom of the ring shadow. Lower lobe predilection. | Change in size of the small air-fluid levels, evident as menisci at the bottom of the cystic lesions, between examinations is virtually diagnostic. |

*(continues on page 186)*

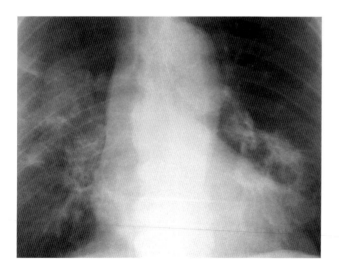

Fig. 9.**24** **Progressive massive fibrosis (PMF)** in coal miner's lung. Besides bilateral perihilar interstitial lung disease and several smaller nodular densities, a larger opacity consistent with PMF is seen in each lung adjacent to a slightly enlarged hilum. The opacity in the left lung depicts massive cavitation due to ischemic necrosis.

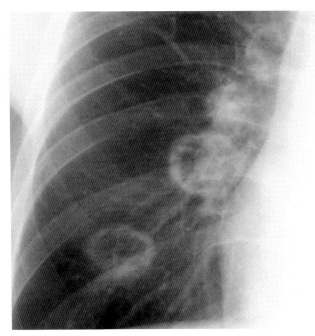

Fig. 9.**25   Wegener's granulomatosis.** Four cavitating nodules are seen in the right lung.

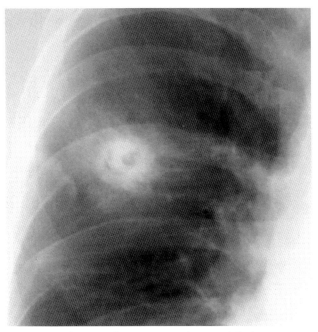

Fig. 9.**26   Pulmonary hematoma.** A dense nodular lesion is seen in the right mid-lung field containing 2 irregular radiolucent foci caused by partial evacuation of the hematoma into the bronchial system.

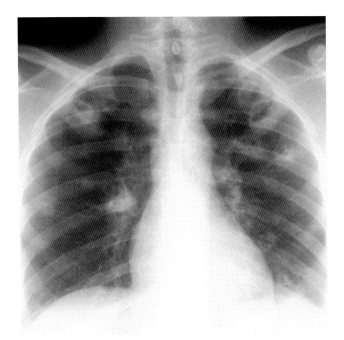

Fig. 9.**27   Septic emboli.** Several round and sharply outlined nodules are seen bilaterally. Most of the nodules have cavitated and some contain air-fluid levels.

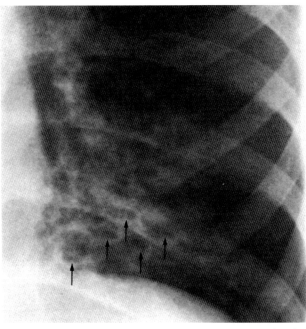

Fig. 9.**28   Cystic bronchiectasis** in Kartagener's (immotile cilia) syndrome (situs inversus with dextrocardia, sinusitis, often with polyposis, and bronchiectasis). Cystic bronchiectasis, some of the lesions with tiny meniscus-like fluid levels at the bottom (arrows), are seen in the left lower lobe.

## Table 9.1    (Cont.) Solitary or Multiple Cavitary and Cystic Pulmonary Lesions

| Disease | Radiographic Findings | Comments |
| --- | --- | --- |
| **Blebs and bullae (Fig. 9.29)** | Cystic spaces greater than 1 cm and confined by thin or even hairline wall that may be incompletely visible. The adjacent lung can be compressed, faking locally a thicker wall. Usually multiple lesions with upper lobe predilection. Pneumothorax is a common complication. | Radiographic evidence of diffuse emphysema may be present. Air-fluid levels develop with infection or, less commonly with hemorrhage. A *solitary bulla* may develop as a sequela of a lung abscess or tuberculosis. It may also represent a bronchogenic cyst whose fluid content has been expelled or is posttraumatic in origin. |
| **Pneumatoceles (Fig. 9.30)** | Solitary or multiple thin-walled cystic lesions commonly associated with staphylococcal pneumonia. | Found in 50% of children with staphylococcal pneumonias. Less common in other pneumonias (e.g., *streptococcal* and *Pneumocystis carinii* in AIDS patients). Results from check-valve obstruction of a communication between a peribronchial micro-abscess and the lumen of a bronchus. |
| **Cystic fibrosis (Fig. 9.31)** | Thin-walled cystic lesions with or without air-fluid levels associated with diffuse, coarse, reticular changes, hyperinflation, and pulmonary arterial hypertension. | Ring shadows are caused by a combination of cystic bronchiectasis, bullae, microabscesses, and honeycombing. |
| **Sarcoidosis (Fig. 9.32)** | Cystic lesions and cavitary nodules are rarely found superimposed on more characteristic diffuse, reticulonodular lung changes. | Mycetomas may occur in these cavitary lesions. (Fig. 9.**33**) |

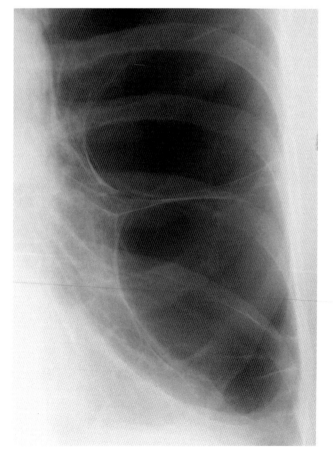

Fig. 9.**29**    **Bullae.** Two large bullae with hairline wall are seen in the left lower lobe compressing the adjacent lung.

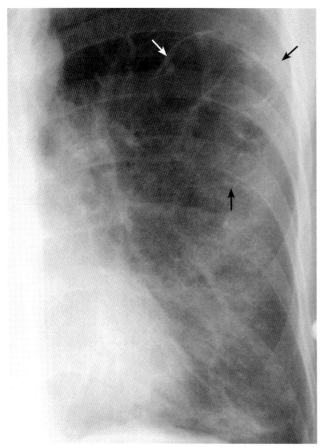

Fig. 9.**30**  **Pneumatocele in pneumocystis carinii pneumonia (PCP).** An irregular cystic lesion with hairline wall (arrows) has developed in this AIDS patient with advanced PCP.

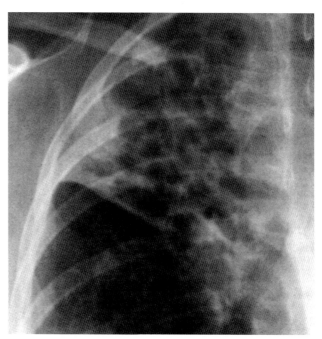

Fig. 9.**31**  **Cystic fibrosis.** Multiple cystic lesions associated with coarse reticular and patchy densities are seen in the right upper lobe. Similar changes were also present in the left upper lobe.

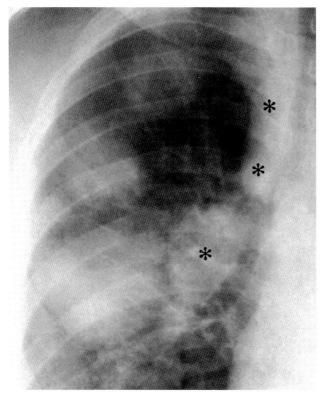

Fig. 9.**32**  **Sarcoidosis.** Relatively poorly defined nodular densities are seen in the right lung. The nodule projecting just beneath the right clavicle has cavitated. Hilar and paratracheal lymphadenopathy (asterisks) is also evident. Similar changes were also present in the left hemithorax.

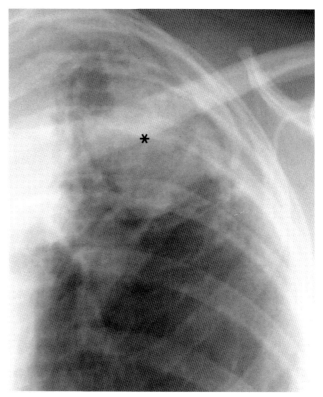

Fig. 9.**33**  **Sarcoidosis.** A cavitary lesion in the left apex containing a large aspergilloma (asterik) is associated with interstitial lung disease including fibrosis (honeycombing) and significant pleural thickening.

# 10 Hyperlucent Lung

The roentgenographic density of the lungs is determined by the absorption of roentgen rays by gas, blood, and tissue. The major blood vessels have a density of 1.0 g/ml, whereas the density of lung parenchyma at total capacity is only 0.08 g/ml. This allows visualization of blood vessels in the lungs without using contrast medium. The density of lung parenchyma increases with the increasing amount of capillary blood and interstitial tissue or fluid. The increase in the amount of contained gas decreases the lung density. A decrease of lung density manifests as increased darkening on the chest radiograph.

The sensitivity of the assessment of bilateral changes in lung density with roentgenograms is limited due to technical variables, variations in the amount of extrathoracic soft tissue, and observer error. CT is able to detect bilateral pulmonary hyperlucency earlier, when plain films are still apparently normal. An apparent *bilateral decrease of pulmonary density* may be caused by three factors or combinations thereof: (1) reduction of the caliber of peripheral pulmonary vessels; (2) reduction of the size of pulmonary hila; and (3) generalized pulmonary overinflation. Four combinations of these changes are possible:

1. *Small peripheral vessels, no overinflation; small hila.*
This combination is indicative of a reduction in pulmonary blood flow and is pathognomonic of usually cyanotic congenital cardiac anomalies with a right to left shunt (tetralogy of Fallot with pulmonary atresia, persistent truncus arteriosus Type IV, Ebstein's anomaly) or of isolated pulmonic stenosis without poststenotic dilatation.

2. *Small peripheral vessels; no overinflation; enlarged hilar pulmonary arteries.*
This combination results from various causes of pulmonary artery hypertension (pulmonary artery stenosis, widespread embolic disease to small arteries, pulmonary arteritis, primary pulmonary hypertension, etc.).

3. *General pulmonary overinflation; small peripheral vessels; normal* or *enlarged hilar pulmonary arteries.*
This combination is pathognomonic of bilateral pulmonary hyperinflation due to an airway disease such as emphysema.

4. *Generalized overinflation of lungs; vascular markings throughout the lungs of normal caliber; normal hilar shadows.*
This combination is pathognomonic of bilateral acute airway disease such as an asthmatic attack or bronchiolitis. The diseases that manifest as combinations 1 and 2 are presented in Chapter 1 and only airway diseases appearing as diffuse, bilaterally hyperlucent lungs, e.g., a general excess of air in the lungs, are included in Table 10.**1**.

*Unilateral hyperlucency* of a lung is easier to perceive than a bilaterally increased radiolucency. However, asymmetry of the roentgenographic density of the two lungs may be due to factors unrelated to lung disease. If the patient is rotated, the density of the lung on which the spine is superimposed will be uniformly greater than the density of the other lung. A similar effect may be produced by scoliosis or by incorrect centering of the roentgen beam. Other nonpulmonary causes of asymmetry of the roentgenographic density are the asymmetry of soft tissues surrounding the chest (e.g., caused by a mastectomy, unilateral hypoplasia, or as absence of thoracic musculature) or a grossly asymmetric thoracic cage. It may also occasionally be difficult to decide whether the side of lower or higher density is abnormal in the case of asymmetric density. Diffuse unilateral alveolar consolidation (e.g., pneumonia), unilateral pulmonary edema, or the effect of pleural effusion on supine film should be easy to exclude as causes of asymmetric density by using the general diagnostic signs of parenchymal disease (see Chapter 20) or pleural disease (Chapter 18).

*Localized pulmonary hyperlucency* may involve the whole lung, a lobe, or a segment. A pulmonary air cyst (bulla or bleb) must be one to a few centimeters in diameter in order to be visible, since the change in density and vasculature can only be compared with the remainder of the lung at that size.

The diagnostic evaluation of localized pulmonary hyperlucency is based on the same variables as is generalized hyperlucency: (1) the amount of air in the involved area, (2) the presence and caliber of blood vessels in the hyperlucent area, and (3) possible changes in the central pulmonary arteries or hilar nodes. The localized decrease of blood flow in the hyperlucent area may cause a compensatory increase of flow in the remaining or contralateral lung. Hilar changes in localized pulmonary hyperlucency may be insignificant or absent in the case of small hyperlucent lesions. When the whole lung is involved (unilateral hyperlucent lung) or when there is compensatory ipsilateral hyperinflation due to lobar atelectasis, the altered caliber or course of the major pulmonary arterial branches or possible hilar adenopathy may provide important diagnostic information.

A fourth important diagnostic variable in localized hyperlucency, the presence or absence of air trapping, is obtained by comparing inspiratory and expiratory films. Lobar air trapping is virtually diagnostic of obstructive emphysema (e.g., foreign body or tumor). Diseases characterized by a unilateral hyperlucent lung or by localized pulmonary hyperlucency and their differential diagnostic features are presented in Table 10.**2**.

### Table 10.1  Bilateral Diffuse Pulmonary Hyperlucency (Overinflation)

| Disease | Radiographic Findings | Comments |
|---|---|---|
| **Chronic obstructive emphysema (Figs. 10.1 and 10.2)** | 1  *General signs of overinflation*: hyperlucent lungs; low, flat, or concave diaphragm; increased posteroanterior chest diameter; increased retrosternal space.<br>2  Limitation of diaphragmatic excursions to less than 2 cm, and air trapping evident by comparing inspiratory and expiratory films.<br>3  Rapid peripheral tapering of pulmonary vessels and their unequal distribution, often with the presence of bullae. Small heart. (*Emphysema with decreased pulmonary markings*).<br>4  Prominent pulmonary vessels of an irregular and indistinct contour and often with cor pulmonale. Bullae uncommon. (*Emphysema with increased pulmonary markings*). | Pattern 3 is common in panlobular emphysema ("pink puffer") and pattern 4 in centrilobular emphysema ("blue bloater"). The "increased markings" emphysema (pattern 4) is often overlooked and regarded merely as chronic bronchitis or recurrent bronchopneumonitis, since signs of overinflation are less prominent. Signs of overinflation may be superimposed and partially obscured by left-sided heart failure. Usually associated with *chronic bronchitis*. In the absence of chronic bronchitis, emphysema may be associated with rare heritable connective tissue diseases (*Marfan's syndrome, osteogenesis imperfecta, cutis laxa*) or with *α₁-antitrypsin deficiency* and predominantly lower lobe emphysema. |
| **Primary bullous disease of the lung (vanishing lung) (Fig. 10.3)** | Bullae (air-filled, thin-walled, sharply demarcated avascular spaces within the lung) more commonly occur in the upper lobes and may grow. There is hyperinflation (as in chronic obstructive emphysema), but no diffuse oligemia of the remaining pulmonary parenchyma. | Primary bullous disease of the lung involves males and is asymptomatic unless the remaining healthy lung parenchyma is severely compressed. Spontaneous pneumothorax from ruptured bullae is common. Bullae are a common feature of chronic obstructive emphysema, with which bullous disease can be fortuitously associated. |
| **Lymphangiomyomatosis** | Bilateral hyperlucent lung may or may not be visible. | Disease affecting woman at ages 20–50. CT is recommended in diagnosis of this disease. |
| **Asthma (status asthmaticus, prolonged asthmatic attack) (Fig. 10.4)** | Severe overinflation of lungs with air trapping. Lowered diaphragm, but it is still convex. The vascular markings throughout the lungs are of normal caliber. Tubular shadows or "tram lines" may represent edema or thickening of bronchial walls. | Between the episodes, the chest roentgenogram is often normal. Severe status asthmaticus and diffuse emphysema can be differentiated by the lack of pulmonary oligemia and the concave configuration of the upper surface of the diaphragm in the former. |

*(continues on page 192)*

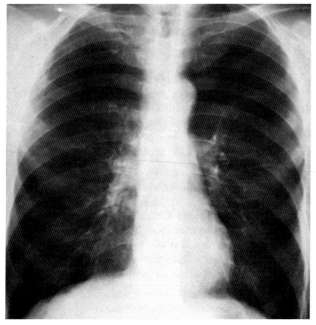
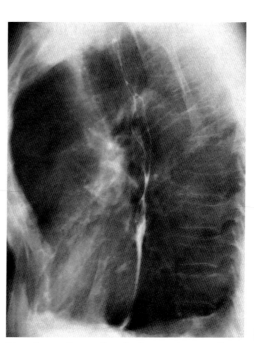

a  b

Fig. 10.**1 a, b  Emphysema with decreased pulmonary markings.** Hyperlucent lungs, flat diaphragm, increased retrosternal space. Rapid peripheral tapering of pulmonary vessels.

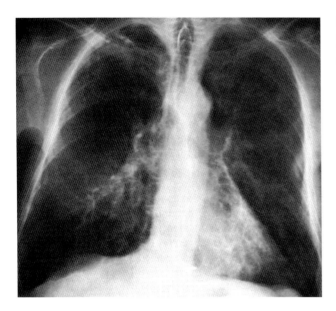

Fig. 10.**2 Emphysema with left-sided heart failure.** General signs of overinflation, prominent pulmonary vessels with indistinct, irregular contours. Small bullae are seen behind the heart. Left ventricular enlargement.

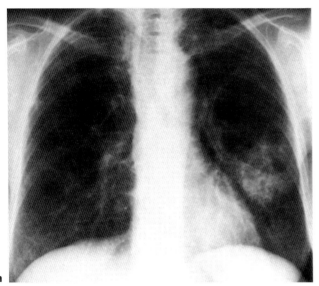
a

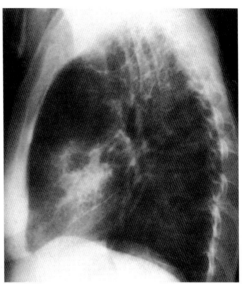
b

Fig. 10.**3 a, b   Primary bullous disease of the lung.** Thin-walled bullae are seen in the mid- and upper-lung fields. The diaphragm is not flattened. Vascular markings in the remaining lung are normal.

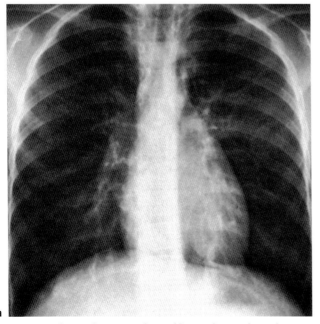
a

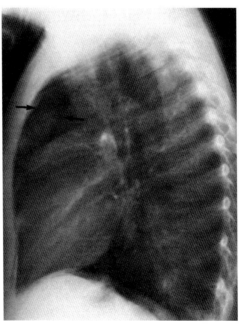
b

Fig. 10.**4 a, b   Asthma complicated by mediastinal emphysema** (arrows). The lungs are overinflated but the diaphragm is concave.

Increased linear markings, especially in the upper- and middle-lung fields, are considered to represent thickened bronchial walls.

## Table 10.1 (Cont.) Bilateral Diffuse Pulmonary Hyperlucency (Overinflation)

| Disease | Radiographic Findings | Comments |
|---|---|---|
| **Acute bronchiolitis (Fig. 10.5)** | Severe overinflation of the lungs may be the only finding. Often accentuated lung markings and small miliary nodules (reticulonodular pattern), particularly in lower zones. Local areas of atelectasis occur in 15%. | Usually a viral infection of small airways. Affects children below the age of three years and adults with a pre-existing chronic respiratory disease. Childhood bronchiolitis may cause unilateral or lobar emphysema (*MacLeod's syndrome*) in later life through *bronchiolitis obliterans*, overdistention and emphysematous destruction. |
| **Diffuse infantile bronchopneumonia** | Diffuse or patchy overinflation. Enlargement of peribronchial lymph nodes. Consolidation usually follows, eventually associated with patchy atelectasis. | This type of bilateral pneumonia is a common complication of *whooping cough*, *measles*, and *influenza*, but is rarely seen in *bacterial pneumonia*. The pattern of roentgen findings may change suddenly. |
| **Cystic fibrosis (mucoviscidosis) (Fig. 10.6)** | Overinflation of lungs. Accentuation of linear markings (bronchial walls). Atelectasis. Recurrent local pneumonias. | Tenacious mucus obstructs air passages. Parenchymal overinflation is largely compensatory, but true emphysema may occur in adults. Excessive concentration sodium chloride concentration in the sweat is diagnostic. |
| **Tracheal or laryngeal obstruction or compression: foreign body vascular ring tumor scabbard trachea tracheobronchomegaly relapsing polychondritis** | All these rare conditions may be visible as overinflation of lungs with associated findings in the trachea (e.g., compression of the trachea and of the esophagus by the vascular ring, collapse of the flaccid trachea during expiration in tracheobronchomegaly) or in lungs (recurrent pneumonias, parenchymal scarring). | *Vascular ring:* The most common tracheal tumors are: *squamous cell carcinoma, adenoid cystic-carcinoma, osteochondroma*, and *papilloma* (especially in children). *Tracheobronchomegaly (Mounier-Kuhn syndrome):* Dilatation of deficient cartilage rings and bulging of intercartilaginous portions. Tracheal diameter is over 3 cm. Affects primarily middle-aged men. *Scabbard trachea:* Flattening of trachea from side to side so that the coronal diameter is equal to or less than two-thirds of the sagittal diameter when measured 1 cm above the aortic arch. Almost exclusively affects men. Emphysema is common. *Localized tracheomalacia* (or stenosis) may be a late complication of endotracheal intubation or tracheostomy. *Relapsing polychondritis* involves cartilage in the ear, nose, tracheobronchial tree and joints |

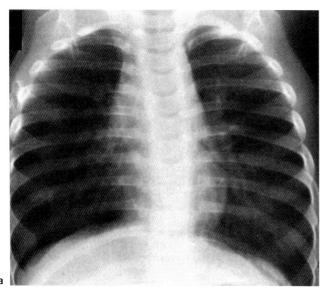
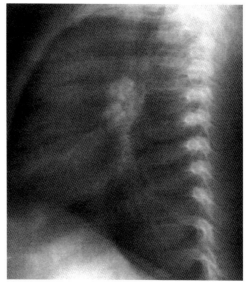

a                                                                                                          b

Fig. 10.**5 a, b   Acute bronchiolitis**, age 1. Severe overinflation of both lungs with flat diaphragm and bulging of lung toward intercostal spaces.

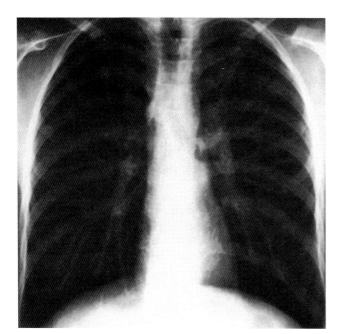

Fig. 10.**6   Cystic fibrosis.** Overinflated lungs contain accentuated linear markings and small patchy infiltrates.

## Table 10.2   Unilateral, Lobar or Localized Hyperlucency of the Lung

| Disease | Radiographic Findings | Comments |
|---|---|---|
| Hypogenetic lung syndrome | Small and, therefore, often hyperlucent right lung, small or absent pulmonary artery, small right hilus. May be associated with scimitar sign (abnormal, curved, broad vein descending toward the diaphragm). | A rare anomaly, often associated with dextrocardia and a mirror-image bronchial tree. The right lung is supplied by systemic arteries (in part or wholly). |
| Absence (proximal interruption) of pulmonary artery | Reduced volume, hypoplasia and increased radiolucency of one lung, usually the right. Small ipsilateral hilar shadow. Absence of air trapping in combined inspiratory and expiratory films. | The anomaly is usually on the side opposite the aortic arch. When on the left, there is a high incidence of associated cardiovascular anomalies. |
| Anomalous origin of left pulmonary artery from the right pulmonary artery | Various degrees of obstructive overinflation and/or atelectasis of the right lung. Posterior displacement of barium-filled esophagus due to interposition of the anomalous artery between lower trachea or the right main bronchus and the esophagus. | Manifests shortly after birth with symptoms of airway obstruction. |
| Congenital bronchial atresia | Overinflation of the apicoposterior segment of the left upper lobe. A smooth lobulated soft-tissue mass (mucus) distal to the point of atresia. Diminution of vascular markings of the affected segment. | A usually asymptomatic, rare anomaly with a characteristic radiographic pattern. May rarely affect other segmental bronchi. Collateral air drift from the anterior segment is responsible for overinflation. |
| Congenital (neonatal) lobar emphysema (Fig. 10.7) | Severe overinflation of a pulmonary lobe, most commonly the left upper, right middle, or right upper lobe. Contralateral displacement of the mediastinum and ipsilateral depression of the diaphragm. Congenital cardiac anomaly in 50 %. | A life-threatening condition that manifests at birth or within a few weeks. Bronchial obstruction is either due to vascular compression or a bronchial cartilage defect, or is unexplained. Since operation is often obligatory, differentiation from other causes of lobar overinflation (foreign body, tumorous bronchial obstruction, congenital, avascular lung cyst, hypoplasia of the contralateral lung, or pneumothorax) should be made. |
| Bronchial adenoma (and other benign pulmonary neoplasms) | Air trapping in *expiration* and possibly oligemia, whereas the volume of the affected parenchyma is usually smaller than normal at full inspiration. Obstructive pneumonitis and atelectasis may follow and are the most common finding. A soft-tissue mass may be visualized. | In most cases, benign bronchial obstruction is complete and results in atelectasis, but occasionally a check-valve effect causes peripheral air trapping. |
| Bronchogenic carcinoma (Fig. 10.8) | A hilar mass with atelectasis is the common manifestation. Air trapping may be present in an expiratory film, but overinflation is rare. | The affected area may be slightly hyperlucent due to diminished blood flow. Overinflation is also a rare finding in *endobronchial lymphomas* and in *tracheobronchial amyloidosis*. |
| Primary tuberculosis | Overinflation of the anterior segment of the upper lobe or the medial segment of the middle lobe. Ipsilateral hilar node enlargement. | Partial bronchial obstruction is caused by lymph node compression or by a granulomatous scar. Atelectasis may follow hyperlucency. |
| Staphylococcal pneumonia | Acute, usually bilateral, pneumonia in a child followed by pneumatoceles, pneumothorax, or pleural effusion. | Common in infants and children. In adults, Staphylococcal pneumonia more likely produces lung abscesses with pleural effusion or empyema. Similar changes may develop secondary to *streptococcal pneumonia*. |

*(continues on page 196)*

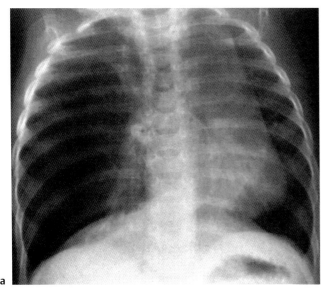
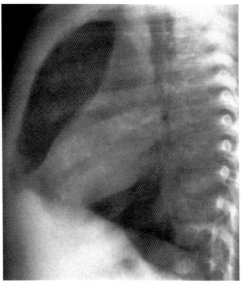

Fig. 10.**7 a, b Lobar emphysema.** Massive emphysema of the right middle lobe, collapse of the rest of the right lung and displacement of the mediastinum. This patient was already 8 months old, but the pattern is similar to neonatal lobar emphysema. No underlying cause was found at operation.

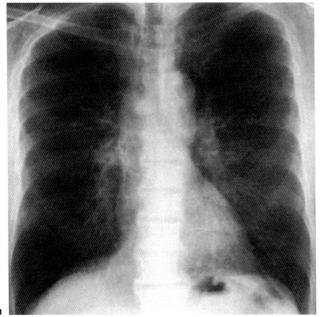
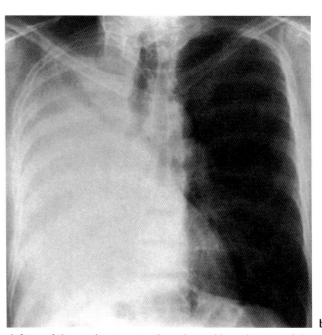

Fig. 10.**8 a, b Bronchogenic carcinoma. a** Slight hyperlucency in the right lung. A subtle density is present in the right hilum. **b** Three weeks later, there is total atelectasis of the right lung, shifting of the mediastinum to the right, and hyperlucency of the left lung.

**Table 10.2   (Cont.) Unilateral, Lobar or Localized Hyperlucency of the Lung**

| Disease | Radiographic Findings | Comments |
|---|---|---|
| Pulmonary thromboembolism (Fig. 10.9) | Widening and abrupt obstruction of a major pulmonary artery. Local oligemia (Westermark's sign). Moderate loss of volume of the involved segment, but may still be hyperlucent due to oligemia. | Pulmonary embolism can cause a variety of radiographic findings, and often no definite diagnostic sign is present. Westermark's sign is useful if films prior to emboli are available. |
| Foreign body aspiration (Figs.10.10 and 10.11) | Air trapping in the expiratory film. Local oligemia may be present. Lower lobe predominance, most commonly on the right side. | Foreign body may be identifiable if radiopaque. |
| Local obstructive emphysema | Changes similar to chronic diffuse obstructive emphysema (Table 1) but localized as assessed roentgenologically. | Function tests indicate generalized disease. Radiographically, lower lobes are more commonly involved. |
| Unilateral hyperlucent lung (MacLeod's syndrome or Swyer-James syndrome) (Fig. 10.12) | Unilateral hyperlucent lung (rarely, the lobe) with normal or reduced volume. Oligemia of the affected lung, small hilus. Air trapping on expiration (diagnostic). | A complication of pulmonary infection in childhood (bronchiolitis obliterans), morphologically similar to emphysema. *Congenital aplasia of the pulmonary artery* is the major differential diagnostic entity. It is not associated with air trapping. |

*(continues on page 198)*

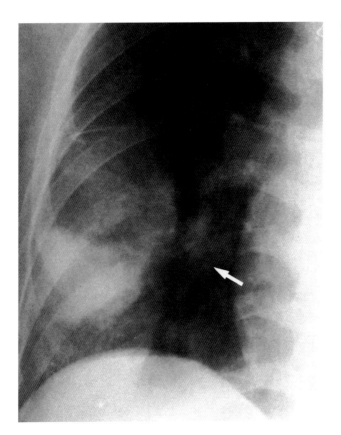

Fig. 10.**9   Pulmonary thromboembolism.** Abrupt obstruction of the right lower lobe artery (arrow), under which there is a hyperlucent, oligemic area. The density lateral to it is a pulmonary infarct.

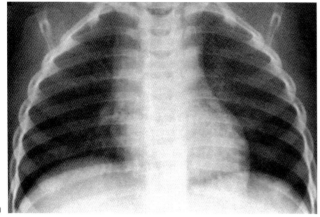
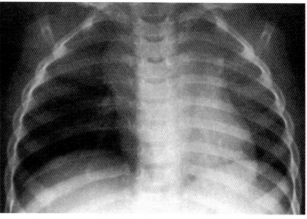

a    b

Fig. 10.**10 a, b    Foreign body aspiration, a** Inspiratory film is normal, but **b** expiratory film shows obstructive emphysema of the right middle and lower lobes, indicating obstruction of the right intermediate bronchus between the branchings of the upper and medial lobes. Note the widening of the mediastinum in expiration, a normal finding in small children.

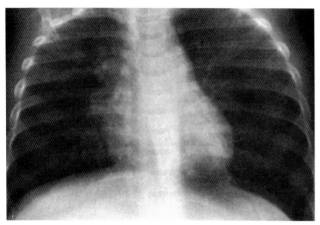
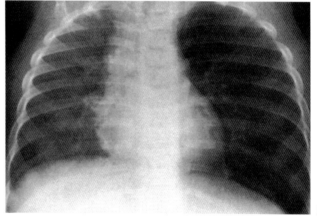

a    b

Fig. 10.**11 a, b    Obstruction of the left main bronchus** (a piece of carrot), **a** Inspiratory film shows minor hyperlucency that is accentuated on the expiratory film (**b**).

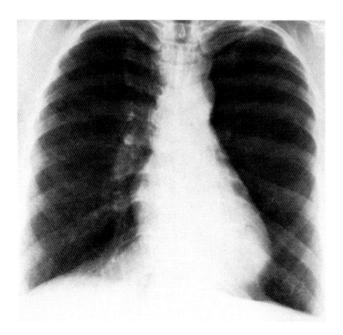

Fig. 10.**12    Swyer-James or MacLeod's syndrome.** Slight hyperlucency of the left lung is caused by oligemia of the left lung and by air trapping (note flat diaphragm).

### Table 10.2    (Cont.) Unilateral, Lobar or Localized Hyperlucency of the Lung

| Disease | Radiographic Findings | Comments |
|---|---|---|
| **Bulla, pneumatocele, bleb (Figs. 10.13 and 10.14)** | Sharply defined, air-containing spaces with hairline walls, can range from 1 cm to the volume of a hemithorax. Vascular markings are absent. Adjacent lung may be compressed. Overinflation and air trapping are usual. | Predominantly unilateral. Unlike in unilateral emphysema, vascular markings are absent. May be a complication of destructive (usually staphylococcal) pneumonia, but may arise de novo. The words bulla, cyst, and pneumatocele usually refer to an air-filled, thin-walled space within the lung. A bleb usually represents a collection of air within the layers of visceral pleura, often associated with the development of the pneumothorax. |
| **Sarcoidosis (advanced pulmonary) (Fig. 10.15)** | Hyperlucency of lungs, reticulonodular pulmonary parenchymal changes eventually associated with blebs, bullae, bronchiectasis, and general emphysema. Cor pulmonale and pulmonary hypertension may be obvious. | Hyperlucent lung in early sarcoidosis is rare. Bronchial obstruction by enlarged nodes occasionally is observed. The other rare cause is the advanced pulmonary fibrosis, which occurs in a minority of cases and is usually bilateral. |

*(continues on page 200)*

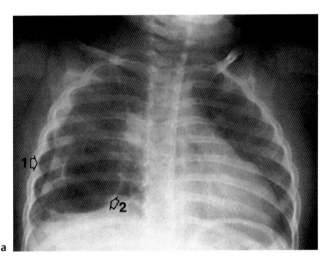

a

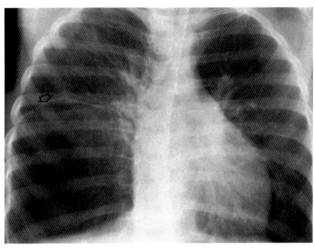

b

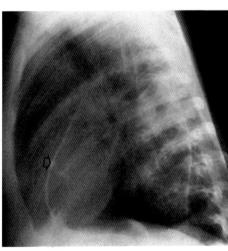

c

Fig. 10.**13 a–c    Pneumatocele and pneumothorax**, secondary to staphylococcal pneumonia, **a** A small right pneumothorax (1) and a pneumatocele in the right lower lobe (2) are seen, **b, c** Same patient, two years later. The right lower lobe pneumatocele has grown into a giant bulla involving one half of the right hemithorax.

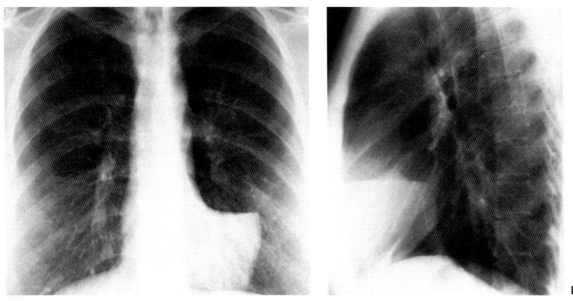

a    b

Fig. 10.**14 a, b    Intrapulmonary cyst.** The cyst compresses the left cardiac margin and in this case produced a peculiar cardiac silhouette, since it contains an air-fluid level.

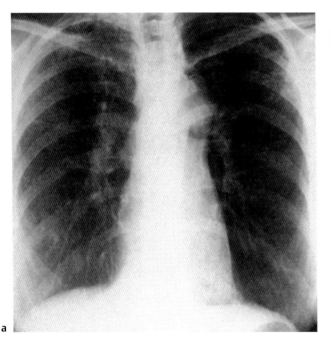
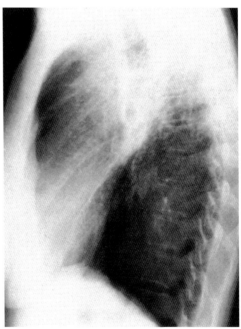

a    b

Fig. 10.**15 a, b   Advanced pulmonary fibrosis with compensatory emphysema in sarcoidosis.** There is shrinking of upper lobes, upward retraction of the pulmonary hili, and resulting emphysema of the lower lobes.

### Table 10.2    (Cont.) Unilateral, Lobar or Localized Hyperlucency of the Lung

| Disease | Radiographic Findings | Comments |
|---|---|---|
| Postlobectomy (post-pneumonectomy) | Reorientation of vessels in the operated lung. Reduced volume of the hemithorax (elevated hemidiaphragm, shifted mediastinum). Distorted or small ipsilateral hilus. Blunted costophrenic angle due to adhesions (late). | Bronchopleural fistula and empyema are common complications, often associated with displacement of the heart and mediastinum to the contralateral side. Excessive fluid accumulation may be due to empyema or delayed bleeding. A decrease in the level of pleural fluid or persistent pneumothorax suggests a bronchopleural fistula. After a *pneumonectomy*, the empty hemithorax is slowly (within 3 weeks to 9 months) filled with fluid. *Herniation of the contralateral lung* is seen often after pneumonectomies. |
| Compensatory emphysema (without surgery) (Figs. 10.16–18) | Collapse of one lobe results in expansion of the neighboring lobe(s). May be produced by bronchial obstruction or any cause of lobar collapse. | Common causes are endobronchial tumors, post-inflammatory lobar collapse, or atelectasis secondary to anesthesia. |
| Pneumothorax (Fig. 10.19 and 10.20) | Absent lung markings. A sharp line of visceral pleura outlines the partially collapsed lung. If unclear, better demonstrated by an expiratory film. Often an air-fluid level (hydropneumothorax or hemopneumothorax) is present. Pleural scarring may produce a loculated pneumothorax. Enlargement of the ipsilateral hemithorax, displacement of the mediastinum toward the contralateral side, often with extensive collapse of the lung, are signs of *tension pneumothorax*. | Spontaneous pneumothorax is most commonly a result of rupture of a subpleural cyst, bleb, or bulla, and is most common in men in the third and fourth decades. It may be a complication of tuberculosis, asthma, eosinophilic granuloma, interstitial pulmonary fibrosis, staphylococcal pneumonia or penetrating trauma. Chronic pneumothorax indicates a bronchopleural fistula. |
| Asymmetric thoracic soft tissues: mastectomy hypoplasia or absence of thoracic musculature | | |

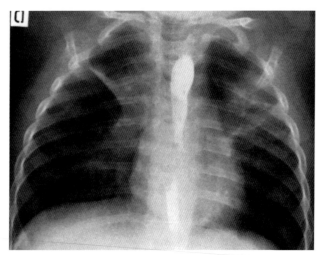

Fig. 10.**16 Congenital stricture of the right upper lobe bronchus** (age 10 months). There is partial collapse of the right upper lobe with expansion and hyperlucency of the right middle lobe. Pneumonia is present on the left side.

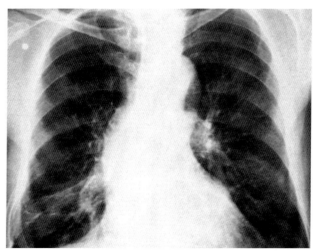

Fig. 10.**17 Healed tuberculosis** with partial collapse and scarring of the right middle lobe, and compensatory expansion and hyperlucency of the right upper lobe.

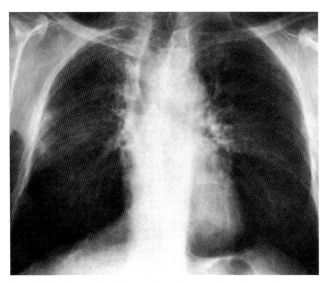

Fig. 10.**18**   **Radiation fibrosis** (carcinoma of esophagus) and partial collapse of both upper lobes with upward retraction of the hili, and compensatory emphysema of the lower lobes.

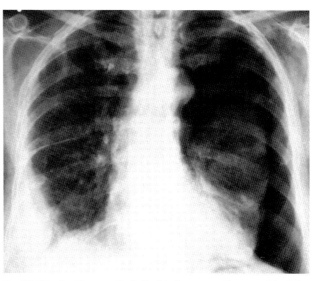

Fig. 10.**19**   **Posttraumatic left-sided pneumothorax** with right-sided pleural effusion and left subcutaneous emphysema. The collapsed lung has an increased density, whereas the rest of the left hemithorax is devoid of lung markings.

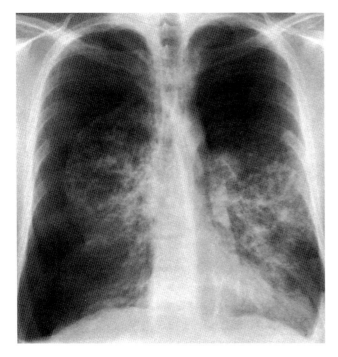

Fig. 10.**20**   Bilateral **pneumothorax** complicating a pneumonia (Pneumocystis carinii and atypical mycobacteria) in an AIDS patient. Hyperlucent pneumothorax surrounds the collapsed and consolidated pulmonary lobes.

# References

Burgener FA, Kormano M. Differential diagnosis in computed tomography. Stuttgart: Thieme, 1996.

Burgener FA, Meyers SP, Tan RK, Zaunbauer W. Differential diagnosis in magnetic resonance imaging. Stuttgart: Thieme, 2002.

Dähnert W. Radiology review manual. 5th ed. Baltimore: Williams and Wilkins, 2003.

Damjanow I, ed. Anderson's pathology. 8th ed. St Louis: Mosby, 1996.

Ebel K-D, Blickmann H. Differential diagnosis in pediatric radiology. Stuttgart: Thieme, 1999.

Federle MP, Megibow AJ, Naidich DP. Radiology of AIDS. New York: Raven Press, 1988.

Felson B. Chest roentgenology. 2nd ed. Philadelphia: Saunders, 1999.

Fraser RG, Paré JAP, Paré PD, Fraser RS, Generaux GD. Radiological diagnosis of diseases of the chest. 3rd ed. Philadelphia: Saunders, 2001.

Goldman L. Cecil's textbook of medicine. 22nd ed. Philadelphia: Saunders, 2003.

Gray HL, Bannister LH, Williams PL. Gray's anatomy. Edinburgh: Churchill Livingstone, 2004.

Kasper D. Harrison's Principles of Internal Medicine. 16th ed. New York: McGraw-Hill Co, 2004.

Keats TE, Lusted LB. Atlas of roentgenographic measurement. 7th ed. Chicago: Year Book Medical 2001.

Keats TE. Atlas of normal roentgen variants that may simulate disease. 7th ed. St Louis: Mosby, 2001.

Kreel L. Outline of radiology. London: Heinemann Medical, 1992.

Kuhn J, ed. Caffey's pediatric Diagnostic Imaging. Chicago: Year Book Medical, 2003.

Kumar V, Cotran RS, Collins T. Robbins and Cotran pathologic basis of disease. Rev Philadelphia: Saunders, 2004.

Meschan I. Analysis of roentgen signs in general radiology. Philadelphia: Saunders, 1973. Two volume set.

Mims C. Medical microbiology. London: Elsevier Science, 2004.

Müller NL, Fraser RS, Coleman NC, Paré PD. Radiologic diagnosis of disease of the chest. Philadelphia: Saunders, 2001.

Reed JC. Chest radiology: patterns and differential diagnosis. 5th ed. Chicago: Year Book Medical, 2003.

Reeder MM. Reeder and Felson's gamuts in radiology. 4th ed. New York: Springer, 2003.

Reeders JW, Mathieson JR. Imaging in AIDS. Philadelphia: Saunders, 1974.

Robbins SL. Pathologic basis of disease. Philadelphia: Saunders, 2002.

Singleton EB, Wagner ML, Dutton RV. Radiologic atlas of pulmonary abnormalities in children. 2nd ed. Philadelphia: Saunders, 1988.

Sutton D. A textbook of radiology and imaging. 7th ed. Edinburgh: Churchill Livingstone, 2002.

Swischuk LE. Imaging of the newborn, infant and young child. 5th ed. Baltimore: Williams and Wilkins, 2003.

Taybi H, Lachman RS. Radiology of syndromes, metabolic disorders. 4th ed. Chicago: Mosby, 1997.

Townsend C. Sabiston Textbook of surgery: the biological basis of modern surgical practice. 16th ed. Philadelphia: Saunders, 2000.

# Index

Page numbers in **bold type** refer to illustrations